Milady's Standard

Hair Coloring Manual and Activities Book:

A Level System Approach

Milady's Standard

Hair Coloring Manual and Activities Book:

A Level System Approach

by Deb Rangl

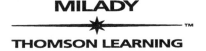

MILADY

THOMSON LEARNING

Africa • Australia • Canada • Denmark • Japan • Mexico • New Zealand • Philippines
Puerto Rico • Singapore • Spain • United Kingdom • United States

NOTICE TO THE READER

Publisher does not warrant or guarantee any of the products described herein or perform any independent analysis in connection with any of the product information contained herein. Publisher does not assume, and expressly disclaims, any obligation to obtain and include information other than that provided to it by the manufacturer.

The reader is expressly warned to consider and adopt all safety precautions that might be indicated by the activities herein and to avoid all potential hazards. By following the instructions contained herein, the reader willingly assumes all risks in connection with such instructions.

The Publisher makes no representation or warranties of any kind, including but not limited to, the warranties of fitness for particular purpose or merchantability, nor are any such representations implied with respect to the material set forth herein, and the publisher takes no responsibility with respect to such material. The publisher shall not be liable for any special, consequential, or exemplary damages resulting, in whole or part, from the readers' use of, or reliance upon, this material.

Cover Design: SoundLightMind
Photographers credit: The Wella Corporation 5-2

Milady Staff:
Publisher: Gordon Miller
Acquisitions Editor: Joseph Miranda
Project Editor: NancyJean Downey
Production Manager: Brian Yacur
Art/Design Production Coordinator: Suzanne Nelson

Printed in the United States of America
8 9 10 11 12 XXX 09 08 07 06 05

For more information, contact Milady, 3 Columbia Circle, PO Box 15015, Albany, NY 12212-0515; or find us on the World Wide Web at http://www.Milady.com

For permission to use material from this text or product contact us at Tel (800) 730-2214; Fax (800) 730-2215; www.thomsonrights.com

Library of Congress Cataloging-in-Publication Data

Rangl, Deb
 Standard haircoloring activities book / prepared for Milady Publishing (a division of Delmar Publishers Inc.) by Deb Rangl.
   p.   cm.
  ISBN: 1-56253-356-8
  1. Hair—Dyeing and bleaching—Problems, exercises, etc. I. Milady Publishing Company. II. Title.
 TT973.R36 1997   97-10089
 646.7'24—dc21   CIP

Contents

Preface

Haircoloring is the largest growing service in the hair industry today. While comprehension and expertise in haircoloring is growing, a continued need for better practical theory and experimentation exists. For this reason, the *Standard Hair Coloring Activities Book: A Level System Approach* helps in the "practice" of cosmetology by providing the latest technology available (at time of printing), plus reference information for continued research.

This book began as a lesson plan for advanced hair color classes for a chain of cosmetology schools. It became obvious early on that advanced hair color theory was desperately needed, as was a better understanding of the basics. After surveying salon owners on various programs, hair color stood out as one of the areas most needing improvement. As the lesson plans grew, something else became obvious, that most advanced color theory and techniques are easily understood by even beginning students when explained in a simple, non-threatening approach.

While teaching the information in this book, other facts became clear. All educators acknowledge that the more practical experiments a student performs, the more confident they become. More importantly, the more a student is exposed to failures or possible problems, the better able that student will be to handle similar situations in the salon environment. This is particularly true of haircoloring. For that reason, this text contains several activities allowing students to practice creating off-color effects, then correct them.

The *Standard Hair Coloring Activities Book: A Level System Approach* compliments and provides additional information to the extensive coverage given Haircoloring in *Milady's Standard Textbook of Cosmetology*. The thorough presentation of haircoloring in the *Standard Textbook* is supported by the information in the *Standard Hair Coloring Activities Book: A Level System Approach.*

The workbook also provides a series of haircoloring activities to enable each student to become comfortable with, and accustomed to using varying techniques to suit the individual client. Instructors will find this book spells out numerous procedures to serve as a teaching aid.

Included in this text are multiple opportunities for students to test their knowledge of color theory.

Deb Rangl

Duluth, Minnesota

About the Symbols Used In This Book

To further aid the student, we've highlighted special areas of the text and represented these sections with three icons:

NOTE: These sections contain particularly noteworthy information that the student may wish to jot down.

TIP: These sections contain extra "inside" information that may save the student time or trouble.

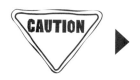

CAUTION: These sections alert the student to potentially hazardous situations and offer suggestions on how to avoid them.

About the Author

Deb Rangl is an international stylist and trainer, with vast experience in all phases of hairdressing. With 20 years experience in cosmetology, she has worked in numerous settings in various roles. As a cosmetologist, Deb has always worked for the upgrading of professionalism, and approached education as a learning *event*. With experience in four different geographic areas in the U.S. including Minnesota, Oregon, Texas, and Florida, and as a former salon owner in Canada, Deb trained with world-class educators before turning her expertise to teaching.

As Director of Programs for four cosmetology schools, Deb has developed curriculum, wrote and directed numerous programs, organized and performed staff training, and developed advanced classes with innovative techniques. Producing fashion shows and competitions helped her generate enthusiasm to motivate students and professional cosmetologists.

Deb gained film experience as an assistant hairdresser on a Hollywood production, and has performed technical and educational work with several color companies. Deb is an experienced platform artist, motivational educator, career coach, and tutor.

Combining years of research while developing curriculum and programs led to a practical depth and understanding for most available color lines. Focusing on both method and client comfort has helped Deb develop standards of excellence that she currently uses in her salon and in training sessions. Marketing is Deb's favorite topic, whether discussing products/services with clients, or delivering a motivational class. It seems to go hand-in-hand with Deb's approach to just about everything, making enthusiasm for new services, ideas, or promotions a standard.

Deb is a member of the National Cosmetology Association (NCA), and the Minnesotas Education Committee, with a major in the Ladies Section and a minor in the Business Section. Education is an ongoing life process for Deb. She has pursued knowledge in many different areas, and is now working toward a degree in business management.

Deb brings her philosophy of life to her career. Caring about people has been the mainstay of her career in the hair industry—that and the art involved with creating a distinctive look for each client she serves. Change makes for creativity, which sparks invention. Deb is constantly assessing her life, career, and goals to shake things up and make things happen. As an owner of two successful salons, one in Canada, and one in Duluth, MN, Deb has incorporated the philosophies both learned and taught to make her business service-oriented and a haven for clients seeking a combination of technical and artistic skills. Sharing her knowledge and experience with others is the most fulfilling side of Deb's career, and one she plans to continually expand through educational classes and writing.

Acknowledgements

The information presented in this text is generally available from most Level System manufacturers. Much of this information was acquired at classes and seminars, over years of research and practicing techniques. A word of caution: marketing can occasionally overcome theory in certain presentations where product promotion is the real goal, not product knowledge. If a claim is *written* it can usually be considered legitimate when distributed by a reputable manufacturer. If a claim is *unwritten,* exaggerated claims are more likely, though not common.

Other useful sources for research were The United States Food and Drug Administration (USFDA), and the Cosmetic, Toiletries, and Fragrances Administration (CTFA).

Information regarding ingredients in hair color products was gathered and verified through numerous sources. Many thanks are due the following:

Mr. Irwin Schwartz, Vice President; Joseph H. Lowenstein and Sons: the main distributor of the raw materials that produce the pigment in hair color for color manufacturers. Mr. Schwartz kindly took time from his hectic schedule to clarify, verify, and define ingredients in hair color, as well as recommend other organizations where research might be extended.

J. Mike Bohen III, Research Chemist; SCRUPLES Professional Salon Products Inc.: for all his help and knowledge regarding hair color, the haircoloring process, and also for referrals for further research. Mr. Bohen has been more than generous with his time and ideas.

Tracy Liguori Lubeley, Director of Marketing; SCRUPLES Professional Salon Products Inc.: for her extensive product knowledge, including in-depth comprehension of the process of haircoloring, her concise presentation techniques, and grasp of information.

Michelle Young, Director of Marketing; AMERICAN INTERNATIONAL INC.: for her help and clarifications regarding the use of Hennalucent® by ARDELL.

Lisbeth Boutang, Operations Manager; Finnish American Publishing: I give special thanks to my friend Lisbeth who used her professional reading and editing skills to help make this work more readable and easily understood to students.

Hazel Christopherson (1919–1997), my mother: who believed my book should be published and wouldn't rest until I submitted it to Milady. She was the best teacher I ever had, wish you could have seen the finished product, Mom.

The publisher would like to thank the following people for their assistance and expertise in reviewing this manuscript: Dee Levin, Philadelphia, PA; Grace Francis, Vista, CA; Phyllis Beesley, Coeur d'Alene, ID; and Carolyn McCallum, Glenarden, MD.

Introduction

"DEAR GOD, PLEASE LET THIS COLOR TURN OUT RIGHT!"

How many times in the past have these words been heard, in the back room or **dispensary** of salons. Okay, I'll be honest. I've used that simple prayer myself many times. I've worked in hair salons in four states and in Canada, managed salons, owned one, and taught beauty school. Everywhere I've worked there has been a fear of tinting hair! Even though I've never been afraid to try anything, I've done a lot of praying!

The biggest reason anyone is ever afraid is lack of knowledge. Timid about attempting haircoloring, stylists often discourage people from trying a tint or color effect. Yes, this strange phenomenon occurs more times than you would think! Stylists have actually talked customers *out* of trying color, resulting in the loss of larger service revenues, retail sales, and eventually the loss of the client, who is disappointed by not receiving the service requested.

Other reasons stylists are afraid to try color or suggest it to clients are: a previous experience that was a disaster, lack of confidence arising from lack of experience, and fear of client rejection with the finished look. Either they don't know what to do with colors or they are afraid to try! *Fear keeps the potentially successful stylist from becoming a true* **technician** *(and rich!).*

SHADE SYSTEM: SOMEWHAT OUTDATED

The original hair coloring system used as a permanent, penetrating tint is called the **Shade System**. It was and still is very effective. The Shade System measures color by its tonal value, such as reds, naturals, golds, browns, and so forth. While many technicians still work with the Shade System, most manufacturers today promote the Level System as easier, and as producing better results.

LEVEL SYSTEM

The **Level System** (the "Thank God" system) totally eliminates the "Dear God" mentality of hair color. Instead of mixing up whatever looks good in the back room, or trying "this" because "that" did nothing, we now have a system that virtually removes all guesswork from tinting hair *and* tells us why! A simple, three-part formula is all you use to determine and achieve great end results.

This text is devoted mainly to the exploration and explanation of the Level System of haircoloring. It includes advanced information usually only provided to the educators who are teaching other professionals. Hopefully this information is presented simply, so it becomes basic color knowledge. A good **philosophy** to follow is: *the more you know, the less you fear.*

The term "haircoloring," as used in the *Standard Hair Coloring Activities Book: A Level System Approach* refers to both the science and art of changing the hair color by using a variety of products and techniques.

The *Standard Hair Coloring Activities Book: A Level System Approach* is designed to familiarize cosmetology students with Level System color and help them understand application and formulation techniques. This workbook should further enhance the *Standard Textbook,* helping you as a student and a professional to achieve a comfort level with haircoloring. It is designed to help make you think and carry through on that thought with "hands-on" practice.

Although most students understand that practice makes perfect, it is perhaps more difficult to understand that in cosmetology, perfect might be a rut. You might learn something to perfection and never go past that point. Hopefully this book will broaden your understanding, first and foremost. Beyond that, it will challenge you to experiment, to think past the immediate moment, and to go forward with confidence, even if you tried something and it failed. One of the best ways to become successful is to know failure. So, when performing any of the activities included in this workbook, keep in mind these are tried and true exercises. If something prevents your activity from working out the way you planned, that's learning! The key to learning these activities is repeating them, especially the ones assigned for strands or models.

Don't be frightened before you begin these activities, but even when you are "licensed professionals" you will have times that your haircolor service does not work out. Be prepared for it! No two human beings are identical, and no two heads are exactly alike. The information included in *Milady's Standard Text* and in this workbook is **theory**, meaning it is scientific information that is supposed to work. The Law of Color is universal, as you perhaps know. However, no laws govern the distribution of genetic blueprints for human hair texture, type, and color. This workbook details the possibilities! If you know the possibilities, and perhaps the limitations, you will, as discussed later in this text, be able to eliminate the fear of failure.

Discover the possibilities—experiment using the activities included in this text, then continue the learning process by applying the concepts in your school clinic work and your work after graduation. Practice makes perfect understanding. Once you understand haircoloring, achieving perfect results becomes easier.

Now that you are hopefully convinced about the value of experimentation, please take heed of this warning. Taking chances is not the same as controlled, planned experiments. As a student, your instructor(s) should always be aware of any projects you plan or are working on, and be available for help if needed. Chemical color products used for experimentation should be applied to human hair swatches; applications may be practiced on manikins or live models. Because strong chemicals are used in preparation, artificial hair will not react the same as untreated, human hair when color is applied.

You will find it useful to gather and prepare the following items as you follow through with the activities included in this workbook:

• Strong cardboard, I ft square

- Natural haircuttings

- 3-inch long plastic ties

- Display tacks

- Fine-tooth comb

- Hair swatches in different levels of color and in different states of condition. For these swatches, **virgin hair** (untreated hair) is considered best. Swatches need to be at least 3 inches in length. Use hair from the same head to make a single swatch about 1/4 inch in diameter when tied at the top.

- When organizing hair for making swatches, turn all ends in the same direction. In wig-making this procedure is known as "root turning." Tie the hair strands together at the end that was nearest the scalp before cutting (Figure I-1). Be sure a swatch contains hair from only one head.

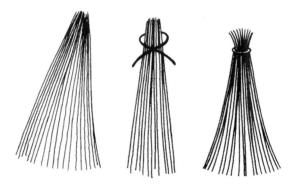

Figure I-1

- Each swatch, however, must be taken from a different head, representing a different level of color, for the results of your experiments to be effective.

- Prepare **natural** hair swatches using a full range of colors—from black to pale blonde. Number hair swatches 1 through 10, number 1 being the darkest, number 10 being the lightest.

1 = dark black	6 = light brown
2 = medium black	7 = dark blonde
3 = light black	8 = medium blonde
4 = dark brown	9 = light blonde
5 = medium brown	10 = extra light blonde

- The hair swatches must be clean before coloring. Once the hair strands are firmly tied, hold at the tied end and swish each in a bowl of warm water containing mild shampoo. Rinse by swishing the cleansed swatch in a clean bowl of water containing a small amount of cream rinse; blot gently between two absorbent towels; comb straight and hang on the "research board" (Figure I-2) beside the number that most closely identifies the natural color.

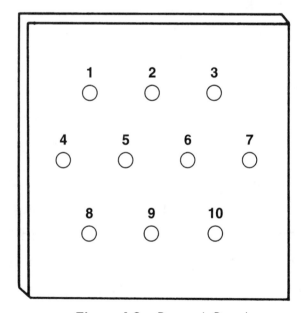

Figure I-2   Research Board

You are now ready to start applying color to the swatches to learn how each product reacts to different hair types and shades. Collect hair samples on a continuing basis so your board can always be replenished after an experimental project.

Throughout this text, you will have various practical assignments and activities to perform. There will be just this one reference to <u>cleaning up</u>, then there will be an assumption that you, as a budding professional, will understand that after each and every activity, you must do the following:

1. **Discard all disposable supplies and materials.**

2. **Close containers, wipe them off, and store them safely.**

3. **Clean and sanitize implements, shampoo cape, and work area.**

4. **Make your work area neat and clean. Fill out and file client card or charting card.**

There cannot be enough emphasis on the value of developing excellent work habits at the start of your career! Your instructors will notice, and once you're in the salon atmosphere, your supervisors, coworkers, and especially clients will notice and come to expect the highest standards from you. It is great to be desired. When clients expect a lot and get it, you are difficult to replace!

As noted above, you will have numerous assignments and learning exercises throughout this text, continuing on to your professional career. SAFETY must be considered first and foremost whenever dealing with chemical products, and hair-coloring products have multiple hazards including:

- Allergic reaction: A pre-disposition or **patch test** is required before each application of aniline derivative tint.

- Alkaline substances: When mixed with hydrogen peroxide they react and cause oxidation, but can also cause heat, and in extreme cases, chemical burns. Clients must be monitored the entire time a chemical is in contact with their hair and scalp. Inquire often as to client comfort, or discomfort. If the client experiences any discomfort, take action immediately. Remove the product, and rinse thoroughly with tepid to cool water, then use a soothing rinse.

- Stains: Not as much a safety risk as a nuisance, but stains can lead to expensive reimbursements if clothing is destroyed. Stains on the skin may require rubbing and/or scrubbing which can irritate skin at worst, and at "best" appear unsightly.

Whether you are performing a haircolor service, or other requested services, it is wise to remember the following:

- Analyze the client's hair. No two clients are alike, and each client must be treated as an individual. You need to observe the characteristics that make up the particular hair you are currently working with.

  Observe:

Porosity	Resistance
Length	Density
Growth Directions	Scalp Abrasions, Irritations, or Eruptions
Scalp Disorders	Texture
Natural Hair Color	Condition
Strength	Elasticity

  Evidence of prior chemical treatments

  Evidence of metallic or vegetable coatings

Many of these conditions may require reconditioning, color removal, removal of coatings or metallic dyes, or postponing the service due to problems with the hair and/or scalp.

Whatever the case may be, discussing, asking questions, and explaining procedures are essential elements of safety *and* client service. These will help with your selection of the appropriate product(s) and application technique(s).

Your best defense with safety precautions is to ask questions regarding your client's background, experience, and previous services. Explain that it is essential for proper treatment and service application to know everything that might affect your service procedures.

Other precautions include:

- Protecting the client's skin at all times. Use a protective cream or petroleum jelly.

- Do not use aniline derivative color on eyelashes or brows, which could cause blindness.

- Do not use any color if scalp has sores, abrasions, etc.

- Never put clients under dryer with color on their scalp unless specifically endorsed by the manufacturer.

- Never leave the client alone in a room—never ignore your client.

- Pay attention to your client—watch for signs of discomfort, scratching, redness, etc.

- Always put client comfort and safety first.

One type of insurance is a release form, which, while not legally binding, will explain that the salon, school, and practitioner believe a particular client's hair is in questionable condition and may not withstand the requested chemical treatment. The release form does help convince clients as to the affects any treatment might have, and your advice regarding the performance of requested services.

Standard Hair Coloring Activities Book

Cleanup is included in all safety precautions, as any product or implements left out and not disposed of properly might lead to problems. Color product left in applicator bottles can swell, even explode.

From the perspective of stylist safety, ALWAYS wear gloves when applying or removing any chemical products! Get used to them, learn to use them without exception, and you will substantially reduce the likelihood of developing chemical sensitivities or reactions.

C H A P T E R

1

The Level System—
What Is It?

In This Chapter You Will Learn:

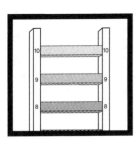

- **The definition of the Level System**

- **Different categories of color**

- **Reasons people color their hair**

DEFINITION

For those who are not clear on what the **Level System** is, the definition is simple—*it is the numerical system of judging color in stages, or numbers, one level being a measure of light or dark in the hair.* The system assigns a number for measuring dark to light without regard to tonal value. Level measures are usually represented by the numbers 1 through 10, each indicating one equal measure (level). However, because there is no universal measurement of a level, one company's level chart may vary from another's. Most of them are similar because there is a limit to the differences between light and dark.

Think of the Level System as being a ladder (Figure 1-1). The first or bottom step is #1 (usually signifying black), with #10 the highest step on the ladder (usually representing very pale blonde). The lower the number, the darker the color; the higher the number, the lighter the color. If you are presently more familiar with the Shade System, three to four shades equal approximately one level in the Level System. The Level System colors always use numbers to indicate **levels** (the measure of light and dark) and letters to refer to **tonal value**, the major contributor of pigment in a particular series. *Example:* 10N means level 10 natural, 9G means level 9 gold, 10S means level 10 silver. Some use more than one letter, indicating contributions of more than one dominant tone. *Example:* GB (gold, beige).

 **Each manufacturer's system of describing individual <u>series</u> differs, but almost all use the same 1 through 10 numbers.**

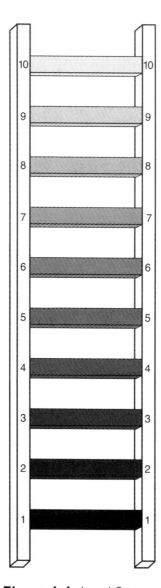

Figure 1-1 Level System ladder

CATEGORIES OF COLOR

The Level System consists of four basic categories of color, as mentioned in the *Standard Text*. These categories are:

- **The B category, dark brown and black:** People born with black or dark brown hair. Levels 1, 2, and sometimes 3 are in the black/dark brown category. They may have some reddish highlights. Their hair darkens with age until it turns gray.

- **The W category, warm brown:** People born with blonde hair that gradually darkens through adolescence. Even before the hair begins to gray the natural hair color loses its warmth and starts to flatten. The hair colorist must keep in mind that the original undertones are still present although the hair has turned gray. These clients can generally wear red tones very well and often request them. They also wear highlights very well. The warm category can include levels from 5 to 10.

- **The L category, light brown:** People born with blonde hair that remains blonde through adolescence. Their hair gradually darkens in their teens to a soft brown color. The soft brown category is usually level 5 or 6.

- **The R category, red:** People born with red hair that remains red throughout adolescence. Their hair gradually darkens or loses warmth with age. The red category usually falls into the levels 5, 6, and 7.

- **Blonde has not been noted as a category.** People with blonde hair, levels 8, 9, and 10, do not usually color their hair until it darkens, although they often add even lighter or brighter highlights for fashion effects. At this point, they are often in the L category.

The Level System is the simplest and most easily performed system of color formulation, providing clear-cut steps to follow with no guesswork. In addition, many level systems contain lower **ammonia** levels than their shade system **counter-parts**, creating predictable, beautiful results.

Please keep in mind that color and light are "seen" differently by each of us—gold to some people is seen as red to others. Many people mistake blue for green, and so on. Pictures of finished colors help a lot during <u>consultations</u>, an important part of the color service, which is discussed in much greater detail later on.

People no longer regard hair as merely a protective fiber! In today's society, hair expresses **image**, a client's fashion and life-style preferences.

Whether your client requires monthly retouches or simply naturalized effects that last for months, color is a repeat business when properly done. To look its best, color must be maintained! With proper consultation, you can customize your color service, catering to every whim and need your clients have. The public continues to spend more time and money to look good. Haircoloring is the most profitable service offered in salons today. Why? A retouch client averages 10 to 12 visits per year! If you hit on the right formula for the client, it equals loyalty! *Clients are very loyal when it comes to color!*

REASONS PEOPLE COLOR THEIR HAIR

So, why do people color their hair?

Let's explore six important reasons:

1. The first and still primary reason people color their hair is to cover or camouflage gray. People want to stay young looking longer; they're living longer and healthier and want to continue to look good! This process began cen-

turies ago, with products using **henna**, metallic-type powders, and other organic substances. The Level System colors enhance or cover gray for healthy, natural results.

2. Equally important to covering gray on our list is the **cosmetic effect** received with a change in hair color. This is especially true in today's image-conscious society. Everyone wants to look his or her best. Presenting the most attractive image really helps to make you successful! Clients care about image! Level System colors produce natural-looking colors that not only enhance hair color, but skin tone as well.

3. High fashion effects are popular for short-term trends, especially with teenagers or people involved in the fashion, music, or arts industries. Although they are more limited to occasional use in most salons, a good color technician will be able to achieve any color desired. Level System produces many **intensified** and fashion tones that shine.

4. Using hair color for contouring or for creating a more **dimensional effect** is helpful in today's tinting procedures. You can make anyone's hair look thicker by correctly matching or complimenting a client's skin tone. Dimensional color makes hairstyles and haircuts look sculptured. It is easy to determine the skin tone level and to add dimension by going up or down 1 or 2 levels. Dimensional coloring is simplified when using Level System 1-2-3 color formulations.

5. **Psychological** boosts are another reason people color their hair. Please don't overlook this area because it has enormous potential for profit and for keeping up the morale and service satisfaction of your clientele. People often need a change, whether drastic or subtle, just to give them a new outlook. *Example:* In the middle of a long, dreary winter, many highlighting

services can be sold. Or, if a client gets a divorce and wants an image change, color is a terrific way to do a makeover. In such cases, it is going to make a *big* difference what color you use. Keep your head; don't do anything too crazy because the client is usually going to regret drastic change. You can create rich, beautiful-looking tones through the Level System's lower ammonia tints.

6. Lastly, an important and profitable part of the coloring business that is often overlooked is **corrective color**. This is when you fix what people do to themselves or (and hopefully you don't get too many of these) what another colorist did to them. It can also include changing a color when the client wants a new look. Often this change will be similar to a corrective color. Corrective colors are usually more time consuming because they often require a color removal service, fillers, and conditioning of the hair. So from a profit viewpoint, corrective color is great business, and made simpler because Level System coloring is usually a three-step process.

IIII➡**ACTIVITY #1:** Role Playing—In-Class Exercise

OBJECTIVE: Enable students to become familiar with identifying and relating to a client's reasons to color hair.

Instructions:

1. Class should be separated into pair groups.

2. Each person in a pair will practice discussing with a partner one or more reasons to color the partner's hair.

3. Each pair will give a brief presentation stating reasons and rationales for coloring each other's hair.

QUIZ

1. Define the Level System.

2. What is the most profitable service in the salon today?

3. Define corrective color. When would a color technician use corrective coloring? Why is this considered a profitable type of color service?

4. What is the primary reason people color their hair?

5. Describe the two effects created by dimensional color.

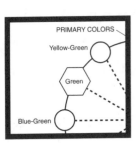

2

The Color Wheel:
It's the Law!

In This Chapter You Will Learn:

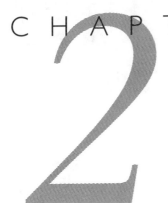

- **Law of Color**

- **Primary, secondary and tertiary colors**

- **Cool and warm colors**

- **Complementary colors**

LAW OF COLOR

You can enhance anyone's appearance with color! Understanding color theory is as easy as knowing the simple **Law of Color** and relating it to *addition and subtraction*. Believe it or not, hairdressers did not invent any of the simple color laws, which trace back to Isaac Newton. Around the same time the apple fell on his head, he discovered that when white light passes through a prism, that light reflects six colors, which make up the colors of the rainbow and are the basis for the **color wheel**. These six colors are:

- Primary colors: yellow, red, and blue

- Secondary colors: orange, violet, and green

Primary colors are colors in their purest form. They are the three strongest and most influential pigments! Any color on earth can be broken down to yellow, red, or blue. Yellow is the lightest primary and is *warm* in value. It is the color hair colorists use most, for it creates the most highlighted effect. Red is the medium-bright primary that reflects more light than the other colors; therefore, it catches the eye first. It is also the *strongest* of the *warm* primary colors. Blue is the darkest, strongest primary. Any time more blue than red or yellow is used in a formula, the color will not only be darker, but less bright. It is the only primary with a *cool* pigment.

Secondary colors are created when two primaries are mixed together. There are three secondary colors. Orange is the strongest *warm* secondary color and is made by mixing yellow and red. Violet is made when red and blue are mixed. It is a *cool* secondary because it is based on the cool, strongest primary. Green, the secondary color with the most *cool* tones, is made by mixing yellow and blue.

When each of the three primaries is placed at the point of a triangle, the three secondaries will fit on points of another triangle (Figure 2-1).

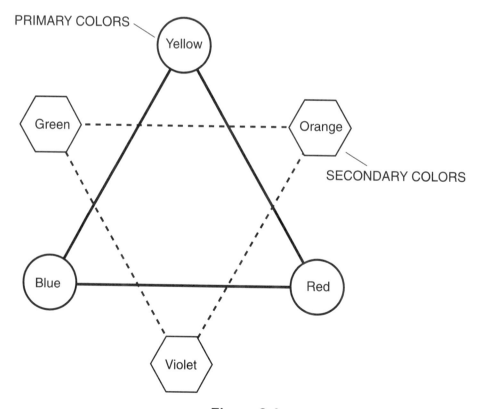

Figure 2-1

This configuration forms the outline of a circle or wheel, hence the term **color wheel** (Figure 2-2).

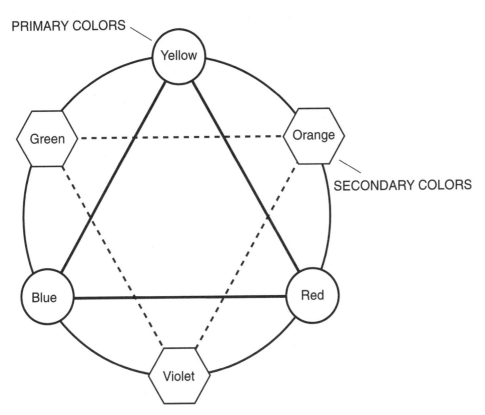

Figure 2-2 Color wheel

The wheel divides into halves—a *cool* side and a *warm* side. Green , blue, and violet are *cool*: red, orange, and yellow are *warm* (Figure 2-3).

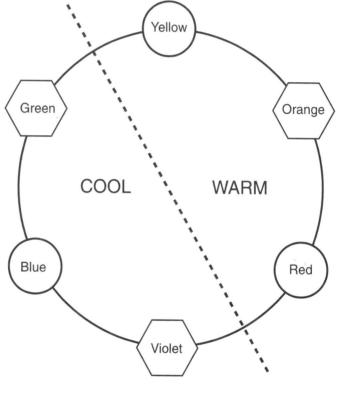

Figure 2-3

Note that each primary color on the wheel is opposite a secondary color. These **opposites** are the true key to success in hair coloration (Figure 2-4).

If colors are opposite each other on the color wheel, they are called **complementary colors**. So what does that mean? **Complementary** means that they complement one another. For example, when yellow is placed next to violet, both colors look their most vibrant and attractive. The same is true with orange and blue or green and red. When two complementary colors are mixed, however, they neutralize or cancel each other, making brown (center of the wheel) (Figure 2-5).

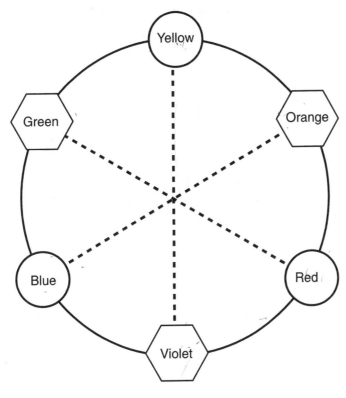

Figure 2-4

The most important fact a color technician needs to remember is the relationship of complementary pairs.

Other colors, called **tertiary colors**, are made when a primary color is mixed with its neighboring secondary color. This combination achieves the most variety and effectiveness in hair coloration, as well as in making any colors on the planet! The most important tertiary colors to cosmetologists are gold (made by mixing the primary yellow with the secondary orange) and blue/violet (made by mixing the primary blue with the secondary violet). These colors also happen to be opposites on the color wheel: therefore, they are complementary. Other tertiaries are red/orange, red/violet, blue/green, and yellow/green. Their placement on the color wheel below shows these colors are complementary (across from each other on the color wheel)(Figure 2-5).

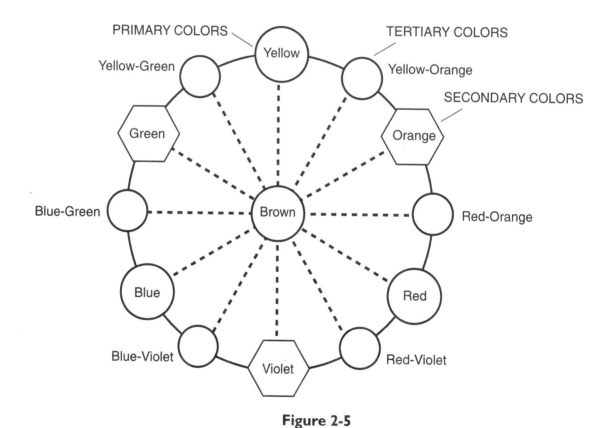

Figure 2-5

All other colors or combinations of colors are called **quaternary colors**. Although these colors are the most varied and widespread, they are not essential in understanding the color wheel because manufacturers describe their products' color bases in terms of primaries, secondaries, or tertiaries.

This theory is known as the **Law of Color**, and it is universally accepted. It is the key to predictable, successful color service.

The Law of Color never changes!

IIII➡**ACTIVITY#1:** Matching

OBJECTIVE: Familiarize the student with the basics of the color wheel.

Instructions: Match the definitions to the appropriate word.

1. color wheel _____   *2.* primary colors _____

3. complementary colors_____   *4.* tertiary colors _____

5. warm colors_____   *6.* violet _____

7. blue _____   *8.* secondary colors _____

9. cool colors _____   *10.* green _____

a. Makes brown when mixed with yellow.

b. The outline formed when primary, secondary, and tertiary colors are placed in proper configuration.

c. Neutralizes orange.

d. Are created when a primary is mixed with its neighboring secondary color.

e. Yellow, red, and orange

f. Colors that are opposite each other on the color wheel and make brown when mixed.

g. Complementary to red

h. Colors in their purest form.

i. Blue, green, and violet

j. Are created when two primaries are mixed together.

||||➡ **ACTIVITY #2:** Labeling the Color Wheel

OBJECTIVE: Provide a visual aid.

Instructions: Insert the primary, secondary, and tertiary colors in the proper configuration on the wheel below, then list the complementary pairs.

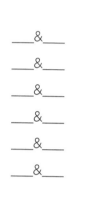

___&___

___&___

___&___

___&___

___&___

___&___

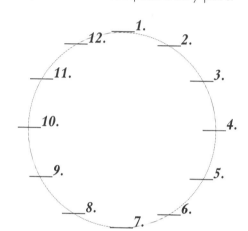

QUIZ

1. Name the three primary colors.

_____

2. Name the three secondary colors.

_____

3. When complementary colors are mixed, they make a shade of what color?

_____

4. What is the universally accepted rule by which all color is measured?

_____

5. List the six major complementary pairs.

_____   _____   _____

_____   _____   _____

CHAPTER

Color: As Simple as Addition and Subtraction!

In This Chapter You Will Learn:

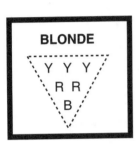

- **Subtraction and addition of color**

- **Understanding brown**

- **Dominant remaining pigment (DRP)**

Here is the first of many important coloring facts many cosmetologists have not learned: When you apply color to the hair, you are adding color. Color + color makes (=) more color, so the hair has more pigment. If the color used is addition only, the hair will often but not always be darker. However, deposit (+ only) tints are frequently used to change tonal value without changing the lightness or darkness of the actual color of the hair. This, by the way, is the least complicated method of tinting hair.

Any time the hair is lightened, no matter how little, you are subtracting pigment. When subtracting color from the hair, one sees an imbalance of natural pigments. Single-process hair color uses both (-) subtraction to remove pigment and (+) addition to replace or add artificial pigment.

"KEEP IT SIMPLE RULES"

1. The three primaries, when mixed in unequal amounts, make brown. If there is more yellow than red or blue, the brown will be light, even beige. If there is more red than the other two primaries, the brown will be warm brown. And if there is more blue than yellow or red, the brown will be dark and cooler looking.

2. Complementary colors turn a brown of some shade of either when mixed. When two complementary colors are mixed, they create the presence of the three primaries in uneven amounts. If you recall from #1, this combination makes a brown color. *Example:* Yellow mixed with violet will make a pale brown because yellow, the stronger color, will dominate the formula. Violet is made from red and blue. When you mix yellow with violet, you achieve a shade of brown. Mixing opposites on the color wheel always results in a "browning out" effect. Simple! Still many stylists don't know this simple rule. They may have forgotten it or didn't know it worked for mixing haircoloring as well as it works for mixing house paint, making clothes dyes, or even frosting a cake!

3. All virgin hair is a shade of brown; it contains all three primaries. Simply, whether hair is *dark brown,* with black being the darkest (the bluest brown, levels 1 or 2–4), *auburn,* (the most warm brown, levels 5–7), or *blonde,* (the most yellow or lightest brown, levels 8–10), the color is an uneven combination of the three primary colors.

Uneven amounts of yellow + red + blue = brown.

Simple! Not only do a lot of hairdressers not know this, they have difficulty accepting it!

Equal amounts of yellow + red + blue = black, gray, or platinum, depending on the level.

Extensive laboratory tests have broken down **melanin molecules** and in *all types* of virgin hair, regardless or race, color, or texture, unequal amounts of yellow, red, and blue are found in each. And, of course, that equals brown.

Seeing Is Believing!

There is a simple way to prove this theory—Play Doh™—yes *Play Doh™*, that colorful clay you played with as a child. Mix a small part portion of yellow and red. You get orange, right? Now take an equally small portion of blue. Mix them all, and what do you get? Brown! Next try a small portion of red and blue. You now get a shade of violet. Mix violet with an equally small portion of yellow, and brown appears, but in a different, lighter shade! Now mix blue and yellow. You get green. Add an equally small portion of red, and brown appears again, although it is a clay or red-dominant brown. All of these little experiments demonstrate that primaries, when mixed in uneven amounts, equal brown. Simple!

MORE "KEEP IT SIMPLE RULES"

1. Balanced color comes when all three primaries are present. When hair undergoes *lightening* (pigment is subtracted), even slightly, there will be an imbalance of the primaries. Color companies always have separate series, with a yellow—or gold—dominant color base, red-dominant bases, orange, blue, blue/violet, green, and naturals. These series often are represented by letters that symbolize their bases. *Example:* G often stands for gold base, R for red, N for natural.

2. The color brown is actually an uneven mixture of three primaries: yellow, red, and blue.

3. In conclusion, very blonde hair is brown with a **dominance** of yellow, red hair is brown with dominant red tones, and black is the bluest brown!

4. To have a balanced, natural hair color, all three primaries must be present. An **imbalance** (lack of any of the three primaries) of primaries leads to an imbalance of the end result.

A simplified example of the **composition** of color molecules in the hair is found in Figure 3-1.

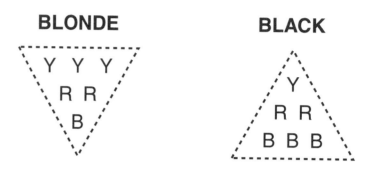

Figure 3-1 The composition of color molecules

When you are lightening color, you are not actually dealing with brown, you are dealing with the underlying or <u>dominant remaining pigment (DRP)</u>, which is usually red, orange, gold, or yellow.

WHAT'S THE DRP?

Cosmetologists with any color knowledge at all understand that warmth is released when you begin to lighten hair. Red and yellow tones will dominate because the first pigment to leave the hair during lightening is blue. If you start with the blackest, most coarse hair and begin to lighten it with **bleach**, you almost immediately see a change. Remember to use a "ladder" to distinguish between different levels of color. At each step, you would see the following colors emerge (Figure 3-2).

To the Human Eye

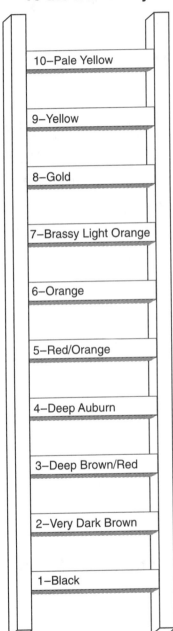

10–Pale Yellow

9–Yellow

8–Gold

7–Brassy Light Orange

6–Orange

5–Red/Orange

4–Deep Auburn

3–Deep Brown/Red

2–Very Dark Brown

1–Black

Under a Microscope

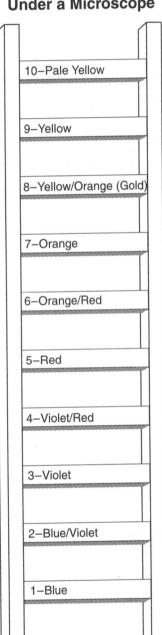

10–Pale Yellow

9–Yellow

8–Yellow/Orange (Gold)

7–Orange

6–Orange/Red

5–Red

4–Violet/Red

3–Violet

2–Blue/Violet

1–Blue

Figure 3-2

Because blue is the first pigment to leave the hair, you would go very quickly into the red zone, which is also the most difficult zone to leave. However, if you use a microscope to observe the same black hair being lightened, you would see a different dominance of pigment at each step or level as shown in Figure 3-2.

SECRETS UNCOVERED!

The second scale opens the Pandora's box of haircoloring secrets that make the color technician an expert. This information is usually reserved for the color manufacturers or the educators of the professionals. A good philosophy is always: *The more you know, the less you fear!* So, if you were to observe the amount of natural pigment remaining in the hair at each level under a microscope, you would see a dominance of blue pigment at Level 1 (black). It makes sense because black hair is really the bluest brown.

- Level 2: very very dark brown, a dominance of blue/violet, which is still very dark but not black, prevails

- Level 3: violet dominates

- Level 4: violet/red

- Level 5: red

- Level 6: red/orange

- Level 7: orange

Level 7, by the way, is the most difficult stage or level to get past, hence the trouble with <u>brassy</u> colors.

- Level 8: dominant remaining pigment is yellow/orange (better known to us as gold)

Standard Hair Coloring Activities Book

- Level 9: yellow

- Level 10: very pale yellow

The **dominant remaining pigment** is the amount of natural pigment remaining in the hair at your target level.

With this knowledge, subtraction (removal or "lift") of hair color, which is usually the most difficult and problematic, becomes easily controlled and understood. An imbalance of natural pigments emerges when subtracting pigment (lifting hair color) because *blue is the darkest primary color.* It is released first, leaving warmth in the hair. This explains why, when lifting many shades (as we often do when seeking lovely highlights and blonde shades), the hair often looks too brassy if the correct formula is not used!

To obtain natural results in haircoloring, simply replace the missing primary at target level.

IIII➡ACTIVITY #1: Play Doh™

OBJECTIVE: Show color mixing.

Materials:

- At least two canisters each of red, blue, and yellow Play Doh™

- Notepaper

- Pen or pencil

Instructions:

1. Using the primary colors of Play Doh™ (red, yellow, and blue), instruct each student to remove from the canister a portion of each color the size indicated:

◯

2. Break this portion into at least four pieces of the size indicated:

○

3. Using one piece of notepaper, draw three dots to form the points of a triangle. Press each of the three primary colors of Play Doh™ to one point of the triangle.

4. Draw three more dots midway between each primary to form a secondary triangle.

5. Take one of the remaining pieces of yellow and mix with red. Identify and position this piece on the proper point of the secondary triangle.

6. Repeat with yellow and blue, then blue and red. Students should now have six colors on the wheel.

7. If desired, continue by mixing another batch of secondary colors. Then combine one-half portions with equal amounts of neighboring primary color to form tertiary colors, positioning each where it should be located on the wheel. (Y + O, O + R, R + V, V + B, B + G, G + V)

8. Using equal amounts, combine blue and orange, red and green, and yellow and violet.

9. Discuss results.

At this point, you should have a color wheel with 12 dots of color representing each of the primary, secondary, and tertiary colors. You should have, by combining the colors in # 8, three different shades and levels of brown.

Which is the lightest?

Which is brightest?

Which is the most drab?

IIII➡ACTIVITY #2: Lighten Black Construction Paper

OBJECTIVE: Demonstrate how pigment is removed and show stages of lightening.

Materials:

- Regular black construction paper

- Gloves

- Bleach formula

- 20 volume developer

- Tint brush

- Timer

Each student may use one piece of paper, or instructor may demonstrate on one sheet.

Instructions:

1. Mix regular powder or oil bleach with 20 volume developer.

2. On regular black construction paper, use a tint brush to daub a streak of bleach across the paper.

3. Observe immediate lightening action. You may choose to blot bleach every 5 minutes, or allow bleaching action to continue undisturbed while class observes the chemical lifting the pigment.

IIII➡ACTIVITY #3: Bleaching Black Hair

OBJECTIVE: Demonstrate underlying pigment and lifting action.

Materials:

- Up to ten 1/4-inch thick strands of black hair

- Regular bleach formula (powder or oil)

- 20 volume developer

- Tint brush

- Gloves

- Foils to place strands on

- Timer

Instructions:

1. Mix regular powder or oil bleach with 20 volume developer.

2. On foils, apply bleach formula to all test swatches.

3. Test every 5 minutes to illustrate lifting action.

4. Identify the different levels as the formula lightens. Try to remove the bleach from one strand for each level achieved. It may be necessary to rinse and reapply fresh formula.

5. Identify the underlying dominant pigments that are visible as the strands lighten.

CHAPTER 4

So What Is Tint, Exactly?

In This Chapter You Will Learn:

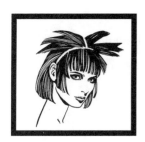

- **Four types of hair color:**

    Temporary

    Semipermanent

    Deposit only

    Permanent, single-process color

There are four types of hair color: temporary, semipermanent, deposit-only, and permanent.

TEMPORARY HAIRCOLORING

Temporary color means exactly what the name says. On normal, healthy hair, temporary colors will not penetrate the hair. They coat the hair; they are usually acidic in chemical composition and are easily removed by shampooing. Temporary color has no lasting quality because it disappears at the first shampooing and will not lighten natural hair color.

Temporary colors (usually **rinses**) are "addition only" and usually last only from shampoo to shampoo. Because temporary colors are nonpenetrating (on healthy hair), they deposit color only to the outside of the **hair shaft**. They are water soluble and therefore affected by weather conditions such as rain, humidity, snow, or even excess perspiration.

Temporary colors will not dramatically change hair color but add highlights or deposit different shades to enhance present colors. The obvious exceptions apply to extremely porous hair, which may take numerous shampoos for color removal, and the color may actually never completely fade from the hair. Temporary colors coat the hair temporarily, do not damage the hair, and often add lustre and conditioning in addition to the deposit of desired colors.

Often the hair nearest the scalp (the most oily and healthy) will be resistant to any type of coating. When applying a temporary color, keep that in mind.

Temporary color is often used to tone or neutralize unwanted yellow in white or gray hair. It is also often used to tone overlightened hair. After a virgin bleach or extreme corrective color, the scalp may be too sensitive for any type of oxidative toner or color. If so, the hair could be temporarily toned with temporary color.

It is, of course, impossible to achieve a color or shade lighter than the base color of the hair being treated. Examples of temporary colors are liquids, rinses, mousses, color refreshers, sprays and crayons, creams, foams, and gels. Most have the same or similar color qualities, but the application for each varies.

Rinses are also called **certified hair colors**, which means they are registered with the **Food and Drug Administration** (FDA). They are considered safe because they are derived from **vegetable dyes** and do not require an allergy or **predisposition test**.

Temporary Colors

(+) only

Main Ingredients:

1. **Pigment**—certified color.

2. **Base**—liquid conditioner, mousse, etc.

SEMIPERMANENT HAIRCOLORING

Semipermanent color is more penetrating than temporary but does not usually leave a **regrowth** line. On normal, healthy hair, semipermanent colors will eventually fade with shampooing.

Many different types of semipermanent hair colors exist, including **traditional** (aniline derivatives that partially penetrate, partially coat) and **polymer** (certified dyes that coat, not penetrate) semipermanent haircolors. These also will not lighten natural hair color.

These varieties of semipermanent hair color are also known as **direct dyes** or "direct coloring" depending on whether traditional or polymer types are being used. The *Standard Text* has detailed information on the polymer type, and this workbook has more on the more widely used method of traditional semipermanent. These dyes are gentle, self-penetrating products that partially penetrate into the outer layers of the cortex, making the *first application* last from four to six shampoos. These products have more lasting qualities than temporary color but are less than permanent.

A common misconception of semipermanent colors is that they will always fade out after four to six shampoos. Not true! This may apply to the first application, but subsequent applications may continue to penetrate further each time, creating a more permanent effect, or a regrowth line.

Semipermanent hair colors are <u>addition</u> only. Semipermanent colors have no lifting capabilities, and they will not lighten the hair, only change tone or brighten existing shades.

Some semipermanent colors will cover gray very well, yet others are not so effective. Semipermanent color is a terrific way to introduce clients to the coloring process. The color will be beautiful and shiny; it will fade gradually, posing no initial threat of regrowth. Usually clients learn to love the extra color, shine, and body and move into permanent coloring effects, which won't fade as easily. Semipermanent colors do not always require mixing before use.

Semipermanent tint can only *deposit* color pigment, but if you want to make the hair all one color, you have to choose a color at the level of the darkest natural color on the head.

Semipermanent Color

(+) only

Main Ingredients:

1. **Pigment**—aniline derivative; patch test required.

2. **Base**—can be shampoo, creme; holds it all together.

3. **Alkaline substance**—can be, but is not always, ammonia; assists gentle, self-penetrating effect of the semipermanent pigment.

4. A **"processing lotion"**—often used, but not hydrogen peroxide.

DEPOSIT-ONLY HAIRCOLORING

Deposit-only color (+ only) happens any time you are making the hair darker or brighter than its natural pigment. This is most often used as color refreshers on gray hair during tint-backs or corrective coloring and reverse highlighting. It is the least complicated type of coloring. The factors to remember are:

- Your base color

- Percentage of gray

- It's also a good idea to add some warmth to the formula when covering gray because the depth of the color may appear too severe without some amounts of gold, red, or both.

- When going two or more levels darker, a filler might be required.

- Color on color always appears darker. If desiring the same level of color, it is wise to actually use a color formula one level lighter to prevent a matte effect.

- Deposit-only hair color will not lighten natural hair color, but adds tonal value.

Deposit-only hair colors use a low volume developer, such as 10 volume, or even 5 volume, to allow for maximum deposit while allowing virtually no lift. The pigment in deposit-only hair color differs from semipermanent hair color, for it consists of both small- and medium-sized dye molecules that allow for greater penetration into the **cuticle** layer. Deposit-only hair colors leave a diffused regrowth line, change the texture of the hair, and last up to 6 weeks. Some of the deposit-only colors on the market today resemble the qualities of semipermanent-type colors and are marketed as such.

Deposit-Only Hair Color

(+) only

Main Ingredients:

1. **Pigment**—aniline derivative; patch test required.

2. **Base**—can be shampoo, creme, gel, etc.; holds it all together.

3. **Alkaline substance**—can be, but is not always, ammonia; assists with the opening of the cuticle, allowing the pigment to penetrate. The percentage of ammonia or alkaline in a deposit-only color is much lower than in a permanent (lift and deposit) color.

4. **Hydrogen peroxide** (developer)—H_2O_2—is responsible for the lasting, permanent quality of the deposit-only haircoloring service. Due to the low volume of the developer, there is little or no lift involved. Hydrogen peroxide will be explained in more depth in Chapter 5, which details the area of permanent haircoloring.

PERMANENT (LIFTING AND DEPOSITING) HAIRCOLORING

The fourth and most important (profitable) color service is **permanent hair color** or **tint**, often referred to as **single-process haircoloring**.

Oxidative color, henna, metallic and compound dyes, and **bleach** are all considered permanent tints.

The <u>Standard Textbook</u> Chapter 12, contains useful information about henna, metallic, and compound dyes. All of these are dyes which coat the hair. Henna is derived from natural materials, while the metallic dyes contain metal or minerals. Compound dyes are combinations of metallic or mineral dyes and a vegetable tint.

While henna might be used professionally, it coats the hair, can build up, and might prevent penetration of other chemicals such as oxidative color or permanent wave solution. Metallic and compound dyes are never used professionally and their presence can react unfavorably with oxidative colors and perms.

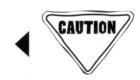

For further information refer to your <u>Standard Text</u>. For information about Hennalucent® as a filler, refer to Chapter 8 of this workbook.

This text deals with the permanent, penetrating tints known as **single-process color**. It involves both subtraction of the hair's natural pigment and addition of synthetic pigment. Permanent color is exactly what it sounds like—it penetrates into the **cortex** of the hair and becomes "locked" in through a process called **oxidation**. Permanent color forever alters the texture of the hair, causing it to swell (gives body). Permanent means the color lasts until it grows out or is cut off. Once hair is permanently tinted, it cannot be made "untinted."

Keep in mind, if you are lightening, you are **subtracting** (-) or **lifting**.

However, in permanent haircoloring (not using bleach), there is also a stage that deposits color pigment into the hair. If you are **depositing**, you are **adding** (+). *Therefore, when you both lighten and deposit color, you are doing both subtraction and addition!* This tint service is the highest in demand, but it is also the most difficult one to do correctly. Still, it is so much easier using the Level System!

Tinted or "pigmented" hair becomes the color lightened (dominant remaining pigment [DRP]) plus your chosen shade.

Understanding the DRP table will make all the difference in your single-process lightening formulas. It is the second contribution in our three-step formula for successful coloration, which will be explained in later chapters.

Permanent color creates a real change in the hair color and texture and always leaves a regrowth.

The single-process tint has revolutionized haircoloring services since its discovery, allowing clients to not only change their natural hair color, but repeat the process as often as the regrowth of the hair requires additional color, *or* any time they choose. Its advantages are natural-looking colors and an ability to be permanent waved effectively without damage to the tinted hair.

IIII➡**ACTIVITY #1:** Color Classifications

OBJECTIVE: Explore each hair color classification.

Materials:

- Seven virgin hair swatches, all from the same head—preferably dark blonde or medium brown having about 20% gray

- One or more tint brushes

- Wax paper folded to make a 20-inch square

- Paper towel (3-folded)

- Seven 1–oz plastic containers (The plastic caps from 1-gallon milk containers make great containers for experiments.)

Products:

- 1–oz temporary color rinse (not more than two shades darker than the natural hair color)

- 1–oz liquid semipermanent hair color (not more than two shades darker than the natural hair color)

- 1–oz liquid oxidizing tint and 1–oz 20 volume peroxide

- 1–oz powdered Egyptian henna and 1–oz water

- No metallic or mineral dyes ever are used professionally! Refer to the *Standard Text.*

- Same with compound dyes. Refer to the *Standard Text.*

Instructions:

1. Using a tint brush, thoroughly saturate one swatch of hair with temporary rinse. Place it carefully on wax paper and allow it to dry.

2. Using a tint brush, thoroughly saturate one untreated swatch of hair with semipermanent hair color. Apply it just as it is in the container.

3. Mix 1–oz of permanent tint (no more than two shades darker than the natural hair) together with 2–oz 20 volume peroxide. Using a tint brush, apply carefully to each strand of an untreated swatch. Place on the wax paper in a warm area and allow it to process for approximately 1/2 hour. (In the absence of body heat, longer processing time is needed.)

4. Mix powdered henna with enough water to make a thin paste. Apply carefully to each strand of hair in an untreated swatch. Place on the wax paper, well away from other projects and allow to process for at least 1/2 hour.

5. At the end of the processing time for each, rinse all product from the hair, add a small amount of shampoo, squeeze it through the hair, and rinse thoroughly. Blot the hair well and allow it to dry on a clean area of the wax paper.

6. Compare and discuss results.

IIII➡ ACTIVITY #2: Matching

OBJECTIVE: Familiarize the student with dominant remaining pigments or end result.

Which DRP must be considered for the following formulas?

A.   Level 6 to level 8 natural   _____   *1.* gold/orange

B.   Level 4 to level 6   _____   *2.* yellow

C.   Level 10 to level 3 natural   _____   *3.* gold

D.   Level 8 to level 10 natural   _____   *4.* orange/red

E.   Level 8 to level 6 red   _____   *5.* orange

List any special problems or requirements with any of the formulas listed above.

_____

_____

IIII➡ ACTIVITY #3: Addition and Subtraction

OBJECTIVE: Further familiarize the student with color formulation.

Instructions:

1.   Using A–E from Activity #2, determine which is subtraction and which is addition.

    A._____   B._____   C._____   D._____   E._____

QUIZ: Types of Hair Color

Identify the following as temporary, semipermanent, permanent, or deposit-only color.

1. Colored mousse _____

2. Single-process color _____

3. Six-week (wash) color _____

4. Henna _____

5. Bleach _____

6. Lasts 4–6 shampoos _____

QUIZ: Ingredients of Color

Outline the main ingredients in each of the following:

1. Temporary color _____

2. Semipermanent color _____

3. Deposit-only color _____

5

Permanent Color

In This Chapter You Will Learn:

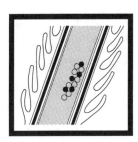

- **Permanent color:**

    Pigment

    Base

    Alkaline substance

    Hydrogen peroxide

- **Working volume**

- **Oxidation: lift and deposit of color**

Permanent haircoloring includes both subtraction (–) of natural pigment and deposit (+) of artificial pigment in one chemical process. The main ingredients are pigment, base, alkaline substance, and hydrogen peroxide.

PIGMENT

Pigment is the tonal value or the dominant hue within a level. Permanent colors contain aniline derivative. Federal law requires that an allergy test be performed before each aniline derivative tint is used. Now, upon reading this, some of you will say to yourselves that aniline derivative has not been used in hair color for many years. Or that the source for hair color products is petroleum distillates. All ingredients are derived from a group of materials that the USFDA defines as a group as being coal tar derivatives. **Aniline derivatives** are oxidative dyes. They are coal tar derivatives, which are derived from coal, not black oozing substances. (The picture that immediately comes to mind.)

There is a broad scope of reference for this group. The reason behind this is that the quality of those materials produced today is *extremely high,* and regulated by very tight specifications. Theoretically, the pigment in permanent hair color is derived from aniline derivatives, or paraminophenyl. Compare that with the actual possible ingredients in different hair colorants listed by the CTFA (The Cosmetic, Toiletry, and Fragrance Association), which number more than 240!

Pigment weight refers to the amount of pigment concentration found at each level of color. Obviously the darker the color, the higher the count of pigment weight. Example: Black (level 1) might have a pigment weight of 240–260. A lightest blonde (level 10) could have as little as 4–6! Deposit colors (darker) usually have much less ammonia required to achieve target color because the pigment weight is so concentrated. For this reason, it is also difficult to achieve more than minimal lift with darker levels due to the pigment weight.

Truthfully, there are many materials used in the production of hair color, and they are considered to be less allergenic than many other products used in cosmetics, fragrances, etc. The materials produced today are so refined, they seem a far cry from the simple "coal tar derivatives" that many veteran color techs remember defined in their textbooks. To illustrate the sophisticated components involved, acetaminophen, a well-recognized safe drug, is made the same way as paraminophenyl.

Most of the raw materials used in hair color are actually colorless molecules called <u>intermediates</u>, which are in a clear liquid form or are coupling agents which combine with the intermediates and an oxidizing agent (hydrogen peroxide) to change their appearance. These small dye molecules possess a color-forming capacity, and it might take as many as six different intermediates to make the color.

The intermediates and coupling agents penetrate into the hair shaft where they oxidize or develop into permanent, insoluble colored pigments that are trapped inside the hair. Level System color manufacturers create wonderful varieties in hair color by combining the intermediates so that they change and form permanent molecules in the hair when mixed with peroxide.

These colors are usually categorized by color series, meaning each series has a predominance of certain colors. For example, <u>Gold series</u> would have a dominance of gold color base, and would help to cover, enhance, and highlight gray hair. Gray is cool and naturally attracts gold. The "N" series usually stands for Natural, meaning balanced with all three primary colors, creating the most effective, natural, gray coverage. A blue-based color would control warmth (orange), and blue/violet would control warmth as well (gold). <u>Red</u> would give a fashion reflection and would also control green or ash casts.

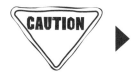

The methodology by which aniline derivatives are manufactured requires that a patch test be performed. These materials have a reported history of producing an allergic response; information regarding the expected number per one million applications is available from the United States Food and Drug Administration. Suffice it to say that any time you use a semipermanent, demi-permanent, deposit-only or a permanent, oxidative color, a patch test is required!

A patch or predisposition test is done at least 24 hours before the color service, and it is applied in the following manner:

A small amount of the color formula that will be used on the client is applied to the skin behind the ear (and covering a small portion of the hair), as well as on the inside of the elbow. The client must be instructed to leave this undisturbed for 24 hours and to let you know immediately if there is an allergic or positive reaction. If the test is negative, you may proceed with the color.

Agreed! This is not a general practice in most salons! It can also be an inconvenience to the client. However, if you have ever witnessed a severe reaction to color, such as bleeding, swelling, or permanent damage of any kind, you already know how important it is to be sure. If the client really wants a color today, but hasn't had a patch test, try a foil or off-the-scalp color. When a client telephones for a color appointment, ask if this is the first time he or she has had color. If the answer is yes, ask the client to come a minimum of 24 hours before the tint appointment for an allergy test. If your client's reaction is, "No one ever made me do this before," be sure and act amazed! Mention how federal law dictates the necessity of a patch test.

Remember whose license is on the line here, not to mention whose good name!

BASE

Base or **color base** can be creme, protein, oil, wax, gel, or shampoo. It's what holds the product together. The better products usually have a cream or gel base, which make for easy mixing, measuring, and application. Many of the finer products have **protein** in their bases, acting as a sled for the pigment to enter the hair. (Pigment molecules adhere to protein in the hair.)

Liquid can either be applied from an applicator or by brush, cream colors must be applied with a brush. Liquid colors contain more ammonia than cream colors, but cream colors often require a higher volume developer for oxidation.

The base determines if a product will be a liquid, gel, or creme.

ALKALINE SUBSTANCE

Alkaline substance is usually, but not always, ammonia (NH_3). It causes the cuticle to swell, allowing for penetration of color pigment molecules and promoting lightening action. You need ammonia to swell the hair shaft. The refined color products available today use lower amounts of ammonia, making for little or no damage and less fading. They also enable the cuticle to close completely after the color process. The ammonia is not a "free" ammonia; it's a derivative (a gas that evaporates quickly). You absolutely need it to open the cuticle. Most of the color products today have a very refined ammonia content that will readily wash from the hair with water.

HYDROGEN PEROXIDE

Hydrogen peroxide (developer)—H_2O_2—is responsible for **oxidation** ($NH_3 + H_2O_2$ = oxidation). It makes the color permanent and must be present for the color to lift and develop, and it makes the color oxidize. First, it reduces (or lifts) the natural pigments (melanin) to reach the desired target level. H_2O_2 is actually H_2O (water) with an extra molecule of O (oxygen). That oxygen is what creates the lift and development of color in the hair.

The higher the percentage of oxygen in peroxide, the more lift you can achieve. Most Level System colors operate with a range of developers from 10 to 40. Ten volume is usually for deposit only, 20 volume for the same level or one level of lift, 30 volume for two levels , and 40 volume for three to four levels of lift. Although volumes vary among the different product lines, all have easy-to-understand scales that will simplify your formulations.

As oxidation occurs, **lift** begins, which is the removal of the natural pigment (melanin) in the hair. Deposit also begins. **Deposit** is a process in which the intermediary color molecules begin joining or locking together to form new color pigment combinations in the hair. With the aid of the H_2O_2, these molecules attract one another and make such large combinations that they become too large to exit the hair shaft and are actually trapped inside. The lift and the deposit occur simultaneously!

Many stylists mistakenly think it is the H_2O_2 that causes the cuticle to open. Not true! The H_2O_2 acts as a **buffer** for the ammonia in color. Its **pH** is actually 2.5 to 4.5. Only when it is released through oxidation does it begin to eliminate pigment.

WORKING VOLUME

The volume of the developer, along with the amount of ammonia in the color, is what determines lifting action. When color product (or any other liquid, for that matter, such as water, conditioner, etc.) is mixed with developer, the H_2O_2 achieves a **working volume (WV)**. WV is the actual volume of the diluted formula. Most color lines use **equal parts** to formulate.

Example: 2–oz color

2–oz H_2O_2

So, if using 20 volume H_2O_2, this formula would have a WV of 10 volume. As the volume of the developer increases, so does the WV. It works on a curve (Figure 5-1).

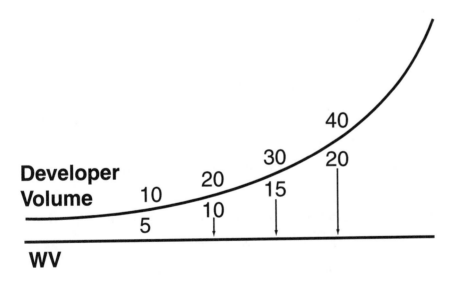

Figure 5-1 Working volume

To keep pace with this curve, many color lines recommend using two times the H_2O_2 for the **maximum lift**, thereby increasing the working volume of the formula.

Understanding working volume helps eliminate the fear of failure. If you need to adjust your volume, or are out of stock, this chart may help you! To arrive at a WV with two different developers, mix equal parts and divide by 2. <u>Example</u>: 20 volume and 40 volume = 60 volume divided by 2 = 30 volume, or 15 WV.

Most product lines include developers with volumes of 10 up to 40 or 60. The highest volume normally used is 40 because any amount above that tends to be less stable. The volume of a peroxide does not determine how *strong* it is, but merely how *long* it will continue to lift. Stabilized H_2O_2 is controlled lifting power: the higher the volume, the more lift. The higher percentage of oxygen in the formula, the more oxidation.

Lower volumes of H_2O_2 and ammonia make for less processing time, less loss of natural pigment, and more deposit. Higher volumes of H_2O_2 and ammonia make for longer lifting or processing time and more natural pigment loss.

Peroxide + Ammonia = Lift and Development of Color. When you mix, you get a funny color (when applied). That's why color is permanent. These two ingredients start out separately, but once they are mixed and applied to the hair, they truly start to oxidize.

During coloring, the H_2O_2 is converted to water and oxygen.

- Water drives the pigment into the hair.
- The oxygen develops pigments.

Once they're developed, pigments enlarge and become trapped inside the hair shaft. Compare it to a mini hydrogen bomb going off in each reaction, causing the intermediates to fuse together. That equals permanent hair color (Figure 5-2)!

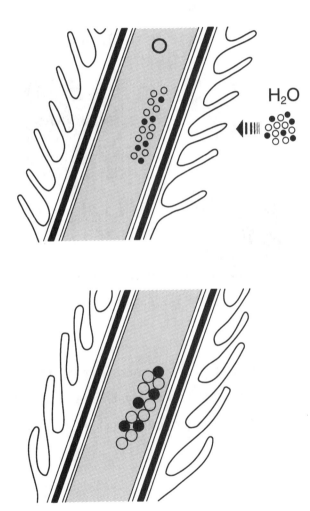

Figure 5-2 Action of permanent haircolor

It is the oxidation process that removes (lifts) melanin! It also deposits color! The colorless intermediates combine to form a compound, which makes the color.

Lift and Deposit Occur at the Same Time. Lift occurs at a more accelerated pace immediately after application, whereas deposit accelerates toward the end (Figure 5-3).

Lift   Deposit

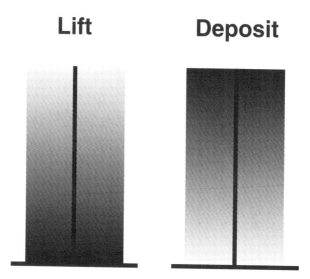

Figure 5-3 Lift and deposit

 **The timing of the process is essential with the Level System. If the product is removed too early, there will not be enough deposit. If the application process is slow, the effectiveness of the lift is impaired.**

GORGEOUS HAIR!

The final result of single-process tint is the total of the hair's natural pigment combined with the product's color molecules. With the Level System use of refined pigments and base ingredients, the result is shiny, healthy-looking hair.

Now that you have the basic knowledge of what color is, how important the color wheel is, and understand *why* permanent tint is the most effective way to color hair, let's move on to the *how!*

For more information on the chemistry of haircoloring, check your <u>Standard Text</u>.

IIII➡ACTIVITY #1: Patch Tests

OBJECTIVE: Demonstrate the procedure for performing allergy tests on clients.

Materials:

- Mild soap

- Same color formula as you are planning to use

- Cotton swab

- Gloves

- Bandages

Instructions:

1. Pair up with a fellow student.

2. Gather required materials.

3. Cleanse area on the inside of the elbow and behind the ear; put on gloves.

4. Apply a dab of the color formula product, mixed using same ratios planned for full head application.

5. Apply bandage to the area to prevent rubbing or staining.

6. Wait 24 hours.

7. Analyze results. If any sign of reaction occurs, color must not be applied.

(For more information, check your *Standard Text.*)

IIII➡**ACTIVITY #2:** Lifting Action of Developer

OBJECTIVE: Demonstrate the lifting ability of different volumes of peroxide.

Materials:

- Four swatches of natural hair no lighter than level 6 (all four should be the same level and tone)

- Level 10 tint, any base

- Peroxide (four different volumes: 10, 20, 30, and 40)

- Tint brush

- Five different containers for mixing tint

- 20-inch square of foil or wax paper

- Paper towel for blotting color

Instructions:

Using level 6 strands of hair and a level 10 color:

1. Mix with 10 volume

   Mix with 20 volume

   Mix with 30 volume

   Mix with 40 volume

Please follow manufacturer's specific instructions for mixing your formulas. Most Level System colors are equal parts, but some are a 2:1 ratio (2 parts developer to 1 part color formula), especially for the high lift formulas.

2. Leave color to develop for the time appropriate for each developer, shampoo each strand, rinse, and dry.

3. Compare results. You should be able to distinguish four different levels of lift by the completion of this activity.

QUIZ: Ingredients of Color

Outline the main ingredients in permanent hair color and describe each:

*1.*_____

*2.*_____

*3.*_____

*4.*_____

CHAPTER

6

Effective Consultation Means Happy Clients and Big Profits

In This Chapter You Will Learn:

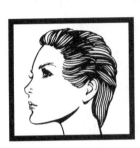

- **Consultations: questions to ask**

- **Observations, considerations**

- **Color portfolio**

- **Base color**

- **Target color**

- **Tea effect**

- **Four rules for natural hair color**

QUESTIONS TO CONSIDER

When you become a professional color technician, consultation becomes one of your specialties! For you to be successful as a colorist, you must know color theory and achieve your clients' desired effects. *More importantly,* you must understand their wants and needs to help them achieve their best images.

How do you accomplish this? It begins by carefully analyzing the client's hair: the texture, condition, porosity, resistance, and percentage of gray. Follow up with an analysis of the individual's skin tone and other physical features. Ask the client many, many questions, such as :

- What effect are you looking for?

- What type of products do you use?

- Are you willing to use the proper products to ensure your hair's condition and lasting color?

- Is your hair colored? (This is one of the most important questions you can ask. Always remember that tint will not lift tint! If color is already on the hair, you must remove it with a **decolorizing** treatment or **stripping shampoo**.)

- Do you want a temporary change or a more permanent one?

- Do you wish a subtle or more dramatic change?

- What type of maintenance schedule are you willing to follow? (Some color techniques are what we refer to as high maintenance, others are virtually carefree.)

- Do you swim? Or use hot tubs? Live in a city with chlorinated drinking water? (All of these will drastically affect lighter hair color and bring out brassy tones in all colors. If this is the case, you will need to recommend suitable products for the type of water the hair will endure.)

- What work environment are you in? Conservative or unrestrained? (This will have a real influence on the client's view of the end result.)

- Are sun exposure, sporting activities, medications, and home demands factors to consider?

The more questions you ask, the better you know your client, so don't be afraid to ask questions!

YOUR COLOR PORTFOLIO

Show the client your color portfolio. What! You don't have one? You don't even know what it is? A **color portfolio** is a book of photographs from magazines or, better yet, from your own clientele file with many examples of gold colors, highlights, reds, mahoganies, plums, blacks, browns, auburns, and all kinds of effects.

This book is a terrific visual aid. Remember that many people "see" color differently. If you "see" what effect your clients like, you will be much more successful (and in higher demand). Keep in mind, most photos of actual haircoloring techniques display more than one color, showing both **highlighting** and **lowlighting**, along with the dimensional effects of **contouring** and **shading**. So, if your client's choice reflects any of those, point out the subtleties of the color. Remember you will have to include them in your color design to satisfy the client. Often, the best technique for initial services in colors includes the use of either **foils** or a **color wash**. Both are more subtle than a complete tint to the entire head.

Whatever the choice is, be sure to outline everything involved—from the color chosen, what is required to achieve that color or colors, cost, and home maintenance to how often the color will have to be maintained. Get a verbal agreement from the client that this service as outlined is acceptable before you proceed. This "precolor" agreement will reassure the client that you understand his or her needs and can achieve them.

BASE COLOR

The color the client has to begin with is called the **base color (BC)**. You need to know exactly what color your client is before you begin to plan a change. *Remember* to ask if she or he has colored hair already. A word of caution—some client's lie! It's hard to believe, but true! Or they think that if they had color 3 months ago, it must be gone by now! Color will not lift color because of the oxidative process. Remember how those color molecules were locked into the hair shaft? Because the tint molecule forms a larger pigmented molecule in the hair shaft, ordinary Level System color does not contain enough ammonia to open the cuticle, enough to allow subtraction of the artificial pigment or allowing for the maximum lift required.

Other things to consider are the categories of color, including the W category, the L category, the R category, and blondes. When formulating perfect colors for your clients, you should consider all contributing factors, the base being your first consideration. The categories of color are important to remember for their dominant tones, as well as for making you think more about each portion of the color process.

Determining a client's base color is essential to the success of every color. This is where you will use the manufacturers' colored swatches that represent each of the color series and levels they provide. Usually, you will want to use the natural series. (Each color company has one, usually symbolized with the letter N.) Try to find the color that matches the client's own color, especially the level of color. If the base is judged lighter than it actually is, you may have trouble lifting to the correct target level.

Eighty percent (yes, 80%!) of the failures that happen with hair color are caused by misjudging the base color. Match your color swatch to the hair at the scalp in the lower crown, the lower nape, and the hairline. This is where the darkest, most resistant hair usually is.

Keep in mind, many clients have more than one base color—usually lighter in front and darker in back. Formulate accordingly!

TARGET COLOR

The desired color you are working for is called your **target color (TC)**. You must know exactly where you are going before you can plan how to get there. Once your client has selected the desired color effect from your portfolio and you have analyzed the texture, porosity, percentage of gray hair, and all other contributing factors, you must use your portfolio to compare with the manufacturers' color swatches to determine your target color(s). At this point you will determine what technique will be required to achieve the desired result.

Your <u>Standard Text</u> has an excellent summary of how to determine whether your client has a cool or warm orientation. This information is essential to the selection of the proper hair color for each client. If a person has warm eyes and skin tone, ash dominant tones in the hair will look harsh and unnatural, and emphasize flaws in the skin. The same is true if a person has cool skin tones and eye color, yet has warm dominant tones in the hair. Understanding and detecting skin and eye tone is a skill that can be perfected only through repeated practice. So practice, practice, practice!

Try to evaluate everyone you know, see, and meet. Determine if their tones are warm or cool. Visualize the perfect color for each person you know or meet. Soon, it will become automatic. When consulting, you will be able to recommend the best color for your client because you have practiced and understand the concept of cool and warm.

OTHER POINTS TO REMEMBER

- How much gray does the person have? Less than 30%, more than 30% but less than 60%, or 60% to 100%? This can make a big difference in your color selection, as well as in the formula you will use.

 **There's an easy way to determine how much gray is in the hair. If it looks more natural than gray, there is less than 30%; if it appears even (salt and pepper), it is 30% to 60%; if it looks more gray than natural, it is more than 60%.**

- If this is a first-time color for someone with more than 60% gray, do not tint to the color the client's hair used to be! Why? The client is used to seeing light hair in the mirror every day. A sudden change is usually very unsettling and noticeable. It's much more effective and attractive starting off two to three levels lighter than the natural (original) color. The look will be more attractive, and it is likely the client will like it so much, that he or she won't want to go darker. Darker than the natural color on a "more mature" person can be harsh and unattractive!

- What is the hair's **texture**?

- **Porosity**?

- **Tenacity**?

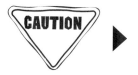 **There may be <u>multiporous</u> hair (hair that has more than one porosity along the strand). Products called <u>porosity equalizers</u> even out or balance the hair's porosity.**

- Will the client purchase retail products to maintain the shine and color depth you give, or is he or she going to use something over-the-counter that will strip the color? This is an important question! If the client will not purchase and use what you recommend, you cannot guarantee the color.

- What type of styling aids does he or she use now? Certain types of fixative products contain so much alcohol they start stripping hair color almost immediately!

- What type of conditioner does the client use? Remember how we are told that an acid-balanced conditioner is great for the hair? And so it is—*unless it's red hair!* Then the conditioner creates what is known as the **tea effect**. Its high acidity will lighten the red color in much the same way a squeezed lemon lightens tea. Red is the largest color molecule and the most difficult to penetrate to the cortex. A very acidic product will shut the cuticle down flat, squirting the red color out!

- Analyze the hair. Does it feel normal, or does it possess a coated feeling?

- If it doesn't feel right, ask. Even if it doesn't feel strange, ask. The only thing that happens when you ask clients questions is knowledge. And that translates into better service!

- Do they take medication (especially high blood pressure or thyroid drugs or hormones)?

- Do they swim in chlorinated pools? Or hot tubs?

- Do they have well water? Mineral deposits are a familiar problem with cosmetologists.

- Is the hair untreated by chemicals, or is it permed or tinted ?

- Any metallic dye? If so, forget coloring over it, which can cause all kinds of disasters!

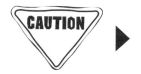

Removal of coating on <u>coated hair</u> is essential to successful coloration. Don't be afraid to counsel, say no, or require conditioning treatments before you provide color services!

A cleansing shampoo before color service is often recommended to remove medicine or mineral buildup. Do not massage, stimulate, or rub the scalp while performing this preliminary service.

Promoting color is a big deal, but you must stand behind your good name. To develop a reputation for excellence, your opinion regarding advisability and feasibility of service must count as the final say when doing a tint service.

Study the haircolor record (consultation form) provided in Figure 6-1.

FOUR RULES FOR NATURAL-LOOKING HAIR COLOR

These are basic concepts that are accepted by color technicians when desiring a *natural hair color:*

1. The hair should be lighter on the ends than at the base of the hair shaft.

2. The hair should be lighter on the surface than underneath.

3. Face-line hair should be lighter than the hair behind it (crown and nape).

4. The darker hair should always be the dominant color. In reverse highlighting, always have more dark hair than light on the head.

Many stylists panic when formulating color. Remember the **fear factor**. They panic because they don't know how to formulate. With most Level System colors, it's a simple three-step formula. Before you learn that formula, it is important to remember or understand that the "how" is much more important to the color

HAIRCOLOR RECORD

Name _____   Tel. _____

Address _____   City _____

Patch Test: ☐ Negative ☐ Positive   Date _____

DESCRIPTION OF HAIR

Form	Length	Texture	Density	Porosity	
☐ straight	☐ short	☐ coarse	☐ sparse	☐ very porous	☐ resistant
☐ wavy	☐ medium	☐ medium	☐ moderate	☐ porous	☐ very resistant
☐ curly	☐ long	☐ fine	☐ thick	☐ normal	☐ perm. waved

Natural hair color _____

	Level (1–10)	Tone (Warm, Cool, etc.)	Intensity (Mild, Medium, Strong)

Condition

☐ normal   ☐ dry   ☐ oily   ☐ faded   ☐ streaked (uneven)

% of gray _____ Distribution of gray _____

Previously lightened with _____ for _____ (time)

Previously tinted with _____ for _____ (time)

☐ original hair sample enclosed   ☐ original hair sample not enclosed

Desired hair color _____

	Level (1–10)	Tone (Warm, Cool, etc.)	Intensity (Mild, Medium, Strong)

CORRECTIVE TREATMENTS

Color filler used _____   Conditioning treatments with _____

HAIR TINTING PROCESS

Whole head _____ Retouch inches (cm) _____ Shade desired _____

Formula: (color/lightener) _____   Application technique _____

Results: ☐ good   ☐ poor   ☐ too light   ☐ too dark   ☐ streaked

Comments: _____

_____

_____

_____

_____

Date	Operator	Price	Date	Operator	Price
____	_____	_____	____	_____	_____
____	_____	_____	____	_____	_____
____	_____	_____	____	_____	_____

Figure 6-1 Haircolor record

technician than it is to the client. Clients are **result oriented**, worrying more about the **end result** or what the finished look will be. They may share some interest as to the how, but what they really care most about are the results! Therefore, your goal when formulating is to have the most effective end result.

IIII➡**ACTIVITY #1:** Create a Color Portfolio

OBJECTIVE: Develop a consulting tool for students to use when working with color.

Materials:

• Photo album

• Outline for desired layout of book

• Pictures from magazines, catalogs, etc., showing blondes, golds, browns, brunettes, multiple effects, trends

• Scissors

• Marker pens for labeling categories

• Construction paper or labels to mark different sections

Instructions:

1. Make outline for the desired layout of the book.

2. Divide album (portfolio) into sections.

3. Collect picture samples of desired effects: blondes, golds, browns, brunettes, multiple effects, trends.

4. Assemble the portfolio in categories to facilitate consultation and selection of colors.

5. Use portfolio for client consultations.

IIII➡**ACTIVITY #2:** Role Playing

OBJECTIVE: To provide practice sessions for students for color consultations.

Instructions:

1. Pair up students.

2. Use color swatches provided by the manufacturer to determine your partner's base color.

3. Decide if hair is cool or warm.

4. Determine level and tone.

5. Determine an appropriate target color.

6. Select the correct formula to achieve that color.

7. Do allergy tests, then perform the color applications in the next class session.

IIII➡**ACTIVITY #3:** "Tea Effect"

OBJECTIVE: Demonstrate the effect of lemon juice (acid) on reddish pigment.

Materials:

• Orange pekoe tea

• Lemon wedge or juice

• Hot water

• Clear mug or glass

Instructions:

1. Brew tea (use clear mug or heat-proof glass to make results visible).

2. Squeeze or pour lemon wedge or juice into tea.

3. Observe results (note the immediate effect of the acidic lemon juice on the reddish tint of the tea).

▐▶**ACTIVITY #4:** Practice Consultations (videotaping or tape recording optional)

OBJECTIVE: Enable the student to perform consultations with ease.

1. Pair up students, practice.

2. Perform consultations.

3. View results; do positive critiques.

4. Repeat as often as class time allows.

▐▶**ACTIVITY #5:** Porosity

OBJECTIVE: Identify multiporous hair.

Materials:

- Two or more swatches of hair that have more than one degree of porosity (the worse the better)

- A container with porosity equalizer

- Wax paper or foil

- Paper towel

Instructions:

1. Separate swatches in groups of two: one for treatment, one for comparison.

2. Use a porosity equalizer on one of the strands.

3. Leave the other strand untreated.

4. Blot product or rinse if required.

5. Compare.

6. Discuss results.

QUIZ

1. Define base color.

2. What is target color?

3. Name the characteristics of cool and warm.

4. What percent of gray will be easiest to cover?

5. Which percent of gray will be most difficult to cover?

6. What is the reaction called when a highly acidic product strips color from the hair?

7. Name the categories of color.

8. What are the rules of hair coloring?

9. Name outside influences that might effect how well a color processes.

10. What is the client's main concern?

CHAPTER 7

Eliminate the Fear!

In This Chapter You Will Learn:

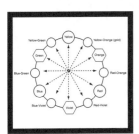

- **Three-part formula for Level System**

- **Contribution of the hair**

- **Contribution of the color**

- **Contribution of the developer**

- **Enhancing and drabbing color**

Always keep in mind the main principle of tinting:

The *dominant remaining pigment* (DRP) at target level *plus* the color you add equals the *end result.*

To achieve the most effective end result, you must consider the contributions of three things:

1. Hair

   a. Base (BL or base level)

   b. Target (TC or target color)

2. Color

3. Hydrogen peroxide (H_2O_2)

CONTRIBUTION OF THE HAIR

- What color is the client's hair now? (Base)

- What color does the client want? (Target)

- Always check the natural color in several areas: the crown, nape, and hairline. Check where the hair is darkest (at the scalp). This is particularly important when lifting.

- Check the percentage of gray.

- Is the base color one level in front, another in back?

Once you have determined what your base is, you must decide: Are you subtracting or adding color, or both?

Addition Is Easy!

If you are doing addition (+) only, the color formula is usually very simple. You use your target color and either 20 or 10 volume developer, depending on each individual manufacturer's recommendation.

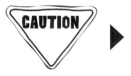

If going more than two levels darker, you may find it necessary to use a filler or repigmentizing treatment.

Subtraction Is the Challenge!

When you subtract (-) color, you must consider your DRP table.

- If you are lifting (-), check the table for the DRP at your target level.

- Decide whether you want to **enhance** (accent) that DRP.

- Or decide whether you want to **drab** (control or neutralize) the DRP.

Example: If you are lifting to a target color of 8N, the DRP at level 8 is OY (gold). *Decide:* Do you want to enhance the gold, making it more gold, or do you want to drab it for a less brassy effect?

If you choose enhance, you would use a color whose base is on the *same side* of the color wheel, adding color to that color.

If you choose drab, you work *across* the color wheel, adding color that neutralizes or drabs the DRP. Remember to use the color wheel to determine what color base you need to use to either enhance (Figure 7-1) or drab (Figure 7-2).

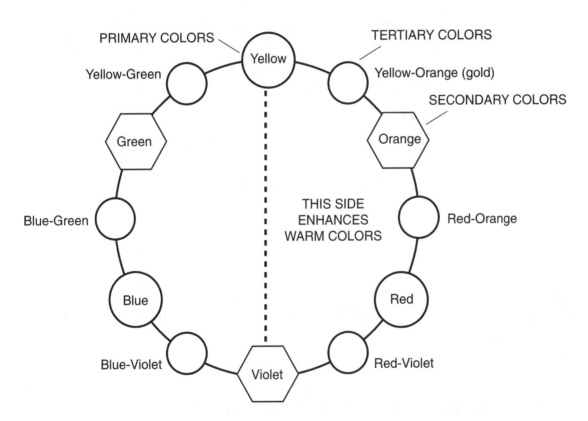

Figure 7-1

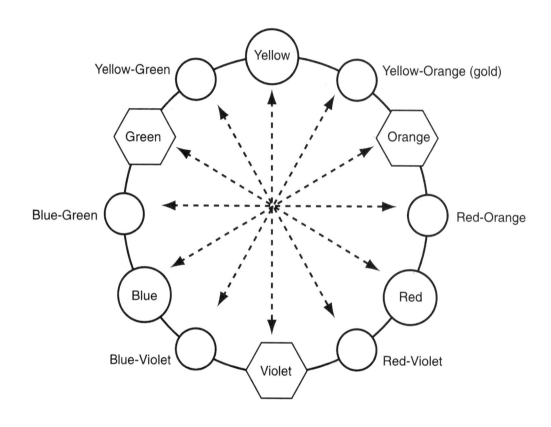

Figure 7-2

 **Complementary colors drab or neutralize each other when mixed.**

CONTRIBUTION OF THE COLOR

The color base you choose becomes your color contribution.

• The level you choose to use is target level for most color lines.

• A good rule of thumb when lifting and drabbing is to *never use your target color.* Why? You need to use a complementary color at target level to drab when lifting!

- When lifting and depositing or depositing, however, you *always use your target level or higher*. It brings the right amount of pigment concentration into your formula to give you the right level of light or dark.

So, the contribution of color is the determination of:

1. Level (whatever your target level is)

2. Color base required (are you enhancing or drabbing?)

CONTRIBUTION OF THE DEVELOPER

The third contribution to a successful formula for desired results is **developer** (H_2O_2).

- Your volume of H_2O_2 depends on whether you are subtracting or adding color. Deposit usually only requires the minimum amount of time for lift; therefore, 20 or 10 volume is the desired volume.

- Each manufacturer has its own "table" for developers, telling you which volume to use to receive the appropriate amount of lift. As your experience grows, you will easily remember and formulate the volume of developer required for each formula.

Not all H_2O_2 is the same! I believe the best results come from using the recommended prescribed H_2O_2 for the color line you use. Remember working volume!

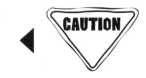

Let's review. End result is the contribution of three things:

1. Hair

   a. Base

   b. Target

2. Color

3. H_2O_2

A Sample Use of This Formula

(For this sample, assume that 10 volume = no lift, 20 volume = 1 level of lift, 30 volume = 2 levels, and 40 volume = 3–4 levels.)

1. Your client has hair contributions of:

   a. Base color—Level 6 natural

   b. Target color—Level 8 natural (desired color)

2. Your color contribution will be level 8 color with a blue/violet base. Consult the DRP table, then determine the DRP at level 8 (OY). Ask yourself if you will be: *drabbing or enhancing* the DRP to achieve your target (drabbing). To determine the color contribution of this formula, you know: 1) You always use your target level and, 2) To *drab,* you must use the complementary color to OY (B/V).

3. H_2O_2 contribution is 30 volume. Your developer will be determined by how many levels of lift you receive for the different volumes.

Your formula for SUCCESS is as simple as 1, 2, 3!

If you always remember that hair color comes down to the contribution of the three things listed above, and if you use the Law of Color with the DRP table, you will have no fear when formulating colors. Most Level System manufacturers use or are compatible with the 1, 2, 3 formula.

Keep in mind the <u>Standard Text</u> information relating to the American Shades System and the European Level System. Most professionals agree that the standard formula today is the three-part formula or a variation of it. The technical knowledge and skills of color technicians will allow them to mix pure-based colors at varying levels in the salon.

IIII➡**ACTIVITY #1:** Cellophanes

OBJECTIVE: Illustrate the "browning out" effect.

Materials:

• Colored cellophanes from a craft store in the primary and secondary colors, cut into 3-inch squares

Instructions:

1. Have students place the complementary colors:

    a. Along side each other to demonstrate contrast

    b. Over one another to show "browning out"

2. Demonstrate effect by mixing: yellow + orange, yellow + red, yellow + blue, etc.

IIII➡**ACTIVITY #2:** Color Wheel Outline

OBJECTIVE: Familiarize students with school's colors and demonstrate how to determine formulas.

Instructions:

1. Provide students with a copy of color wheel, (using yellow, red, blue, gold, red/orange, and blue/violet) or allow time for each student to outline a color wheel.

2. Using the information from the manufacturer reference or according to its base and level, insert each color in the proper alignment on the color wheel.

3. Practice determining what color to use when enhancing or drabbing.

IIII➡**ACTIVITY #3:** Test Swatches

OBJECTIVE: Practice achieving off-colors.

Materials:

• Strands from light to dark

• Various color formulations

Instructions:

1. Using strands from light to dark, try to make a strand with each of these colors: orange, yellow, brassy, silver (ash), violet or mauve.

2. Discuss formulas used and end results.

IIII➡**ACTIVITY #4:** Corrective Color

OBJECTIVE: Practice achieving brown or neutral colors from off-colors.

Instructions:

1. Using the strands from Activity #3, try to achieve a neutral or brown.

QUIZ

1. Name the three contributions involved in achieving your end result:

_____

_____

_____

2. What contribution involves the client's base and target color?

_____

3. Which side of the color wheel do you use to drab a color?

_____

4. Which side of the color wheel do you use to enhance a color?

_____

5. What is the third contribution in successful color formulation?

_____

CHAPTER

Repigmentizing, Otherwise Known as Filling

In This Chapter You Will Learn:

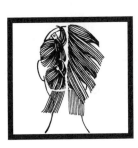

- **Repigmentizing or filling**

- **When to fill**

- **What filler to use**

WHY FILL?

What is a filler? A **filler** can be described as color pigment concentrate, without mixing with peroxide first, so it does not provide lift. Most manufacturers recommend colors from their gold-, orange-, or red-based series for repigmentizing or filling. Occasionally, conditioners or reconditioners are used for filling. These build the hair's integrity, enabling the color molecules to process correctly.

Neutral Hennalucent® is also occasionally used as a "fiber filler" to plump hair and fill the cuticle. Neutral is used as opposed to a colored product because the transfer of translucent powder resin becomes part of the fiber but does not adjust the fiber in any way, nor add any color tones. Therefore, this product is best used *following* an oxidative color to seal or trap the color, and give the hair more body and shine. This product does not block chemical penetration, or react adversely with chemicals as other henna products might.

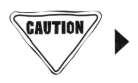

While henna might be used professionally, it coats the hair, can build up, and might prevent penetration of other chemicals such as oxidative color or permanent wave solution.

Why use fillers? When your tints are lacking in one or more of the primaries, you will probably need to fill the hair, or **repigmentize**, to replace the missing primary.

1. If you're going two or more levels darker, you will often need to repigmentize for a successful color.

2. Fadage problems—If your tints fade drastically between services, repigmentizing helps, whether you are lifting the client's color or depositing.

3. Tonal value is off—If your tint has a strange or undesirable cast, it improves your chances of achieving a wonderful end result to fill the hair before coloring, as the filler gives the color more "color" to hold.

Always remember, when going darker, your colors automatically have a lot of blue pigment just to make the levels drop, so the fillers you need to concentrate on are yellow, orange, and red.

- For natural colors, when filling, you always need to use one level lighter for the stronger warmth.

- If you fill during your color, you must fill at the level you are targeting or one level lighter.

Most colorists prefer applying the filler first, then blotting the excess and applying the color formula right over the filler.

WHICH FILLER?

How do you know what filler to use?

- Refer to the manufacturer's technical manual for first reference.

Standard Hair Coloring Activities Book

- Otherwise, a good rule of thumb is to go with the warm tones in the next level up from your target color. If your target has a lot of warmth, go with a filler that has a lot of gold and orange.

Why would you need a filler with a high lift color?

Your ends might have faded drastically, creating a damaged effect or a two-tone color. Use a light gold first to fill, or as directed by the manufacturer of your tint product.

Occasionally on very porous hair, the filler is first protein conditioner, then color filler.

⫸ACTIVITY #1: Comparison Swatches

OBJECTIVE: Familiarize student with the principle and necessity of filling or repigmentizing.

Materials:

- Enough pairs of matching pre-lightened swatches to demonstrate (Once again you need the same color swatches in groups of two. One swatch will be for your application, the other for comparison.)

- Filler formulas recommended by individual manufacturers or a medium gold and a medium red

- Wax paper or foils

- Containers for mixing formulas

- Tint brush

Instructions:

1. Divide strands into two groups.

2. Determine:

   a. Base color   *b.* Target color   *c.* Fillers needed

3. Apply filler to half the strands; leave others without filler.

4. Allow to process according to manufacturer's directions.

5. Blot excess.

6. Mix target colors.

7. Apply each target color to a filled strand and one without filler.

8. Process for recommended times (same time for filled and nonfilled strands).

9. Shampoo, rinse, and dry.

10. Compare results.

QUIZ

1. Another name for filling is _____ .

2. Why fill when doing high lift color?

    _____

3. Give three reasons to fill when depositing color:

    _____

    _____

    _____

4. You should always use a filler when depositing _____ or more levels.

5. When you fill, you replace the missing _____ .

CHAPTER

9

Bleaching—Big Bucks, Not Big Fear!

In This Chapter You Will Learn:

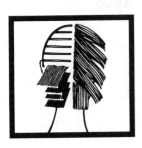

- **Lighteners**

- **Color removal formula**

BLEACHES OR LIGHTENERS

Different lightening products (bleaches) on the market are great for different effects. Your *Standard Text* discusses the basic description for lighteners, and the three types used by cosmetologists. If you are doing on-the-scalp lightening, the one recommended is usually a creme bleach because it doesn't dry as quickly with the body heat. It also has buffers, which allow for more boosters. Off-the-scalp (foils, weaves, frosts, etc.) usually call for **powdered bleaches**. They lift more quickly, and their consistency facilitates application. **Creme oil bleach** is available for on-the-scalp lifting but is considered slower and milder. Whichever you decide to use, remember bleach is a strong chemical and must be used with care and safety.

Double-process tinting is a service where the hair is first prelightened with a bleach formula, then toned with a pastel or fashion shade. This service is discussed at length in your *Standard Text*.

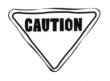

▶ **Always wear gloves when performing lightening services.**

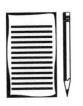

▶ **To wear hair color extremely light (platinum) it must be lightened every 10 to 14 days. The simplest and most effective way to get a very light, white look is to <u>retouch</u> often!**

If your clients are hesitant about having their lightening services performed this often, and who can blame them, keep in mind that past 1/4 inch away from the head, the natural pigment will not lighten as quickly due to the lack of body heat. Apply to the shaft first, then to the scalp area, which will lighten much more quickly.

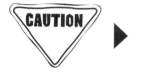

▶ **Treat bleached hair like the precious, easily damaged treasure that it is!**

▶ **Recondition with protein after every bleach service, if not after every shampoo! Advise clients about the at-home maintenance that is required with a great light look.**

Many clients will opt for the high lift look or a foiled, highlighted effect instead of the constant maintenance of bleaching. Once a client is hooked, however, you can take the money to the bank, as long as you take care of the hair, scalp, and the client!

Keep in mind the power of positive, professional vocabulary! "Bleaching" hair sounds less professional, cheaper, and dated. You are performing a lightening or highlighting service!

In case you are already thinking that it's "too much trouble" to lighten on the scalp, many world-class competitors and internationally renowned stylists love hair that has been lightened with bleach and toned (referred to as **double-process** or two-step coloring). The reason for this preference for lightened or high lift colored hair is the pliability and flexibility of the hair. The hair shaft is expanded due to the chemical reaction, creating lots of "body" for easily molded hair.

Although it is possible to lighten hair from very black to very light, it is not usually done for the following reasons:

- More pigment in the darker hair substantially increases processing time and potential damage to the hair and scalp.

- Most people with dark hair do not lighten through 10 stages because of the rapid appearance of dark regrowth and subsequent maintenance.

In the hair industry this process is referred to as "high maintenance" hair.

- Skin tone of people with extremely dark-colored hair usually looks better with medium light, not extremely light hair.

The procedures for lightening do not vary much from school to school or manufacturer to manufacturer. The procedure in the *Standard Text* is typical for a lightener application procedure.

For retouches, apply the product to the shaft and ends <u>only</u> if necessary to lighten more or if there is off-coloring on the strand. If it appears absolutely necessary to remove off-color tones or brassy bands, dilute your lightening formula with <u>conditioning</u> shampoo, then follow your lightening service with a deep reconditioning treatment. Repeated use of high ammonia products is extremely hard on the hair and may easily cause severe damage or breakage!

Be careful! Always recondition after any lightening treatment!

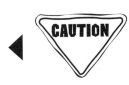

COLOR REMOVAL FORMULA

The **color removal formula** is also known as a **decolorizing** or **stripping shampoo**. Although different types of stripping shampoos work basically the same, a good one for:

- Removing color from hair to be tinted lighter

- Removing excess deposit from hair immediately after tint

- Helping **presoften**

- Achieving a maximum of one to one and a half levels of lift

is:

2–oz H_2O_2

2–oz bleach (1–2 scoops)

1–oz shampoo

1–oz conditioner

This formula is applied at the shampoo bowl, and it must be applied very quickly and evenly. A recommended use is a tint brush and bowl, applying in broad sweeps of the brush. Because the formula works very quickly, care must be taken and the formula must be monitored from the entire time it is on the head. The formula can be strengthened or weakened by decreasing the amounts of shampoo and conditioner used, or by diluting with more of the same. When this product is applied, the conditioner and shampoo act as buffers for the bleach formula, making it far easier on the hair and scalp.

Standard Hair Coloring Activities Book

Although this formula seldom causes discomfort, always be aware that it is a decolorizing (bleaching) formula; therefore, it has a higher pH than most tints.

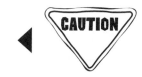

Remove by using **tepid** water and conditioning shampoo. Always recondition after lightening the hair!

IIII➡**ACTIVITY #1:** Create Green or Silver Hair

OBJECTIVE: Increase student's confidence in color formulation.

Materials:

- Several yellow-blonde strands, either bleached or natural (enough for group participation)

- Tint formulas using level 8, 9, and 10 with blue base in the formula

- 10 or 20 volume developer

- Wax paper or foil

- Gloves

- Tint brush

- Containers for mixing formulas

Instructions:

1. Using level 8, 9, and 10 blue base colors, prepare formulas of each.

2. Apply to strands.

You may also use blue/violet base on white-blonde strands.

3. Check frequently, watching for ash green or silver to develop.

4. Remove when green or silver-purple color develops.

5. Observe results.

6. Discuss technique for correcting these off-colors.

IIII➡ **ACTIVITY #2:** Color Removal

OBJECTIVE: Demonstrate color removal and color correction.

Materials:

- Swatches from Activity #1

- Containers for mixing formulas

- Tint brush

- Foils or waxed paper for applying formulas

- Ingredients for color removal formula

- Gloves

Instructions:

1. Use strands from Activity #1.

2. Mix color removal formula.

3. Apply to strands.

4. Check frequently (every 30 seconds) because color lifts very quickly with this formula.

5. When off-color effect is lifted, shampoo, rinse, and dry.

6. Discuss results.

QUIZ

1. List the formula for color removal.

2. What lightening formula works best?

3. Should you recondition lightened hair?

4. What is the simplest and most effective way to maintain a very even, light blonde effect?

5. Explain the application for the color removal formula.

6. Name the three types of bleach available.

7. Which type is usually used on the scalp?

8. Which type is normally used for foils, weaves, and frosts?

C H A P T E R
10
Corrective Haircoloring

In This Chapter You Will Learn:

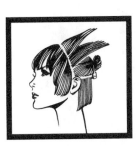

- **Things to consider**

- **Two safe assumptions**

- **Categories of corrective color**

PROFITABILITY

Corrective colors are usually the most easily charged-for service for the following reasons:

- You usually need multiple steps to "fix" the color.

- Conditioners are essential.

- Fillers are almost always required.

- Your expertise as a colorist is challenged *and* valuable.

- Often these services are one-time only. Possibly more than one visit will be required, but the client knows most of the initial expense was for correction.

Corrective coloring can be controlled and safe providing you follow certain rules and actually "look for trouble." In other words, question the client regarding previous treatments, then ask yourself these questions:

1. Is the hair in good or bad condition?

2. Are the client's expectations realistic?

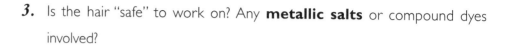

3. Is the hair "safe" to work on? Any **metallic salts** or compound dyes involved?

4. Have I thought of all the possibilities, and do I have a plan of action?

As with regular color <u>formulations</u>, you must consider the three contributions for the end result:

1. Hair

   a. Base

   b. Target

2. Color

3. H$_2$O$_2$

If the hair is damaged, or even questionable, you are much wiser to proceed slowly. Do not take chances. Recondition as much as you think is necessary before proceeding. If the integrity of the hair is compromised to the extent that it is weakened, breakage may occur. Just as important, color may not adhere to protein-deficient hair, but fade or wash out quickly.

Whenever you do corrective coloring, two assumptions are safe:

1. You will almost always need to use a filler or repigmentize the hair.

   Fillers:

   a. Help to equalize excessive porosity.

   b. Deposit color to faded ends in the absence of developer.

   c. Make streaking and off-color less likely.

   d. Produce natural-looking tint having uniformity and shine.

To determine what filler to use: Follow the manufacturer's advice, or go with a filler that has deep red plus gold for levels 1 to 5; orange for levels 6 and 7; and gold for levels 8 to 10. The intensity of the filler should be determined by the level of your target color.

2. You will need to recondition the hair.

    a. Prior to your corrective color service, reconditioners help the pigment adhere to the hair.

    b. After your corrective color, reconditioners help "lock" in the pigment, making it fade less.

    c. Reconditioners allow you to proceed—with caution!

TYPES OF CORRECTIVE COLORING

Corrective coloring is usually done for these reasons:

1. Fix what clients or others have done.

2. Create extreme changes in image.

3. Tint from lighter hair to darker, natural color (tint-back).

4. "Strip" or remove color treatments before lightening to achieve lighter levels.

5. Correct off-colors (green, silver, purple, blue, brassy, and so forth).

Fixing Mistakes

Unfortunately, many clients "play around" with color at home. Some are lucky; many are not. Although as professionals we may talk until we're blue in the face about reasons for them to let us do their hair, human nature tells some clients "you can do it yourself." They do, and sometimes get it *really* wrong: brassy gold instead of sandy beige, green instead of ash blonde, black instead of their own soft brown.

Your response to these predicaments might be, "I'll do what I can. I know my colors and won't give up until you have a nice color again." If done properly your clients will swear by your skills when finished! A goal for corrective color: Keep expectations reasonable, then knock their socks off!

Most clients are so desperate when needing a terrible color fixed, they practically become groupies when you deliver a lovely, natural, healthy-looking color. Plus, they expect to pay more because they made the mistake in the first place!

Image Change

You can warn your clients, "This service costs more. I do this, this, this, and this to ensure your color looks as great as possible." The procedure for an extensive image change varies depending on the client, but it usually involves multiple steps, and each step involves time. Time, in turn, is charged for.

Tint-Backs

Tint-backs are services that return the client to her previous color or a darker color. They almost always require fillers and usually require conditioning.

Color Removal or Stripping

A color removal service is almost always followed by a toner or tint, and for a good reason. The color remover has a higher pH, which opens the cuticle of the hair. An oxidizing tint, on the other hand, fills that cuticle and can act as a conditioning treatment with its lower pH. The oxidation will lock in the color and reflect more shine. A toner or tint also requires reconditioning and often fillers on porous ends and can also require more than one tint formula for different areas.

Correcting Off-Colors

This procedure often includes a color removal treatment, conditioning, and filling porous ends, depending on the base color level and target color.

IIII➤ACTIVITY #1: Tint-Back Formulations

OBJECTIVE: Further expose students to color formulation in corrective coloring.

Instructions:

1. Using swatches from Activity #2, Chapter 9, do tint-back formulas for the following: level 6 natural; level 7 gold; level 4 natural; level 4 red.

IIII➤ACTIVITY #2: Tint-Back

OBJECTIVE: Learn effective application of corrective techniques.

Materials:

- Swatches from Activity #2, Chapter 9

- Formulas from Activity #1 above

- Tint product

- Peroxide

- Containers for mixing products

- Tint brush

- Wax paper or foil

- Gloves

- Fillers if required for specific formulas

Instructions:

Using the formulations from Activity #1 above:

1. Apply formulas.

2. Check every 5 minutes.

3. Remove when processed to desired color.

Remember full deposit often requires maximum processing times.

QUIZ

1. List reasons for corrective color.

2. Prior to a tint-back, what services might be required?

3. When using a filler, what color do you use?

4. Correcting off-colors often includes

   a. _____

   b. _____

   c. _____

5. To correct level 9 ash to a level 8 natural, what do you use?

11

Methods of Application

In This Chapter You Will Learn:

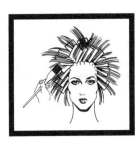

- **Procedures:**
    Brush
    Method D
    Method L
    Retouch
- **Color removal (shampooing)**
- **Weave/foil applications**
- **Lightener applications**

The methods used for **application** are many and varied. Several modes of application are equally adequate and professional.

Be advised that you should:

1. Make it look as though the client would have difficulty trying to copy your procedure at home. (Brush application)

2. Make your application as neat and professional as possible.

3. Find a method that is easy for you to master and use efficiently. In other words, get it on fast!

Keep in mind, color begins developing the moment it is mixed with the developer, so you have to be very competent with your applications.

CONSULTATION AND PREPARATION

Begin all color services with client consultation! Then:

1. Most salons today prefer having their clients change to a tint gown for the process. It's much more practical, not to mention safer when it comes to any spills that might occur. If a customer has a stain on his or her clothing, it is not the customer's fault—it's yours. You alone are responsible for making certain the proper procedures and precautions are taken.

2. If you do not have gowns at your disposal, make sure you protect the client's clothing with a towel. At all times make sure the cape is pulled out from the chair to protect clothing.

3. Preshampoo! Use a **clarifier** and really get down to clean hair! Comb through hair and dry under a cool dryer to avoid scalp irritations.

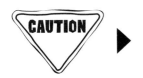

Don't scrub or stimulate the scalp before a chemical treatment—just lightly apply the clarifier making sure it absorbs into all the hair.

4. Next, place a towel on the outside of the cape around the neck and clip. (You may, on occasion, have salon owners or managers who don't want you to use too many towels—honest!). Whatever the policies and procedures followed, try to rate customer comfort as your first and utmost consideration.

Keep in mind: detail = service = profit!

5. Before mixing the color, use cream around the edges of the hairline (on skin only) to prevent stains and irritations. The only exception is with light blondes because the pigment weight will not allow for staining of the skin.

6. Section in quadrants (fourths).

   a. **Part** from middle ear to ear.

   b. Part down the center of the head.

   c. Clip out of the way.

Put on your gloves! Always use gloves, or eventually your hands will develop sensitivities to products not to mention how awful those stained hands look!

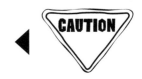

7. Mix color right before applying to use the full development time. Most manufacturers want you to put the H_2O_2 in first, then the color. For lifting tints, you should mix only enough formula to apply to one section at a time.

8. Start applying where?

   a. If you're going darker, start in the lightest area (usually the front).

   b. If you're going lighter, start in the darkest area (usually the back).

As a rule, when applying color, outline each section first, except right on the hairline edges. Do it quickly. It will aid you by showing the outline of your work. Don't apply right on the hairline hairs at first because they're so fine they will "grab" darker.

BASIC PROCEDURES

The following is a normal tint application using a brush procedure found to be effective:

1. Begin *applying* at the top of the head.

2. *Slant* your sections up toward the front to accommodate the round shape of the head.

3. *Use* very small section lines (1/8 inch for retouches and 1/4 inch for shaft applications).

4. *Start* 1/2 inch out from scalp for virgin lightening or reds.

5. *Apply* from roots to ends with virgin hair going same tone or darker.

6. *Rest* the handle of the brush on the tips of the forefinger and middle finger; hold the brush in place with your thumb.

7. *Rotate* the brush between thumb and finger to use the tip of the handle to make diagonal **partings**.

8. *Draw* a line to your thumb.

9. *Grasp* the sectioned hair between thumb and forefinger.

10. *Push* excess hair downward with the brush handle still flat to separate the strands.

11. Then *lift* the strand away and out with tension, then upward.

12. *Dip* brush in color formula.

13. *Scrape* the product from the back side of the brush.

14. *Rotate* the brush in your fingers and *apply* to the regrowth from the top of the regrowth in one continuous motion.

Standard Hair Coloring Activities Book

15. If regrowth is less than 1/4 inch *use* the edge of the brush, drawing tips of brush along the subparting, working the color into the scalp.

16. *Repeat* until finished.

Some reminders may be helpful:

- Be careful! Don't **overlap**!

- Dip your brush in the color formula for each section application.

- Remove any excess color from the skin around the hairline as soon as your application is completed. The more care you take during and immediately after application, the easier the color removal will be!

- Lift the hair out from the scalp to assist the oxidation process.

- If you are applying to the shaft or ends, coat the brush more liberally. (These areas are more porous and require more product.)

You should still use one side only of the brush for neatness; hold the hair on your outstretched palm and work the color into the hair on your palm. After coating all the hair, comb the product from scalp to ends, or as indicated by the process you require.

Your color is complete when the desired color is reached (usually when the regrowth matches the shaft and ends).

Virgin Hair

There are basically two accepted methods for regular applications of tints to virgin hair.

METHOD D is used to darken hair. It may also be used when lightening the hair less than one level.

1. Using 1/8-inch partings, apply to the scalp area on the entire head.

2. Immediately apply to the shaft and ends, using 1/4-inch partings.

3. When processing is complete, shampoo.

METHOD L is used to lighten the hair one level or more.

1. Using 1/4-inch partings, apply starting 1/4 to 1/2 inch from the scalp up to porous ends.

2. Process until the shaft is almost exactly the color desired.

3. Using 1/8-inch partings, apply a fresh mixture to the scalp area and to the ends depending on the extent of porosity at ends.

4. When the scalp area is the same color level as the shaft and ends, remove the color.

Retouch Application

For a normal amount of regrowth, using 1/8-inch partings, apply to all the new growth according to the brush application procedure. Process until the color is developed, then **blend** to shaft and ends with color, a shampoo cap, or apply a semipermanent color to the shaft and ends as a color refresher. When the regrowth and shaft and ends match in color, remove the color.

 **If you choose a bottle application, be sure you keep your sections tiny and keep all the product either on the client's hair or in the bottle.**

Removal Procedure

Most color will basically lift itself from the scalp if removed properly. The following technique will work with any tint.

1. *Moisten* hair slightly with water. Thoroughly *massage* the hairline area first, then the rest of the head, using small amounts of water while working (emulsifying) the product.

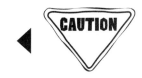

If too much water is initially used with the product removal, the base might gel on the scalp, making removal more difficult.

◀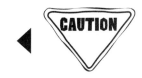

2. After the product is completely lifted by massage, *add* water gradually while massaging until the water runs clear.

3. At this point, before shampooing, *check* the nape area, dampening your used tint towel with tepid water to remove any runaway tint from the nape, ears, etc. Then *wipe* the neck of the shampoo bowl before proceeding with the shampoo.

4. *Shampoo* vigorously with the proper shampoo formula for color-treated hair to remove any color residue.

5. *Rinse* thoroughly.

6. *Shampoo* twice!

7. *Apply* conditioner to the hair and rinse.

For reds, use the higher acid pH conditioner, not low pH, to avoid the tea effect.

◀

WEAVE AND FOIL PROCEDURES

Because **weave** and **foil** techniques are so predominant in today's salons, every colorist needs to have skill in the application of these techniques. Frosts are being replaced with more accurate and professional foils with weaving and foiling techniques. These techniques not only intrigue the client and look as though they are more artistic and difficult, they are nearly impossible to duplicate at home. Here are some suggestions for great streaks or weavings.

Weave Procedure

After consultation, plan color(s) to be used and your pattern. *Example:* Use two colors, a blonde and a medium red, to add highlights. Alternate two blonde weavings with one red to have a golden blonde highlight, two red with one blond for a more strawberry blonde effect, or one medium lift light blonde, one darker golden blonde, and one thin slice one or two levels darker than the client's own color. This gives movement and dimension to the hair (Figure 11-1).

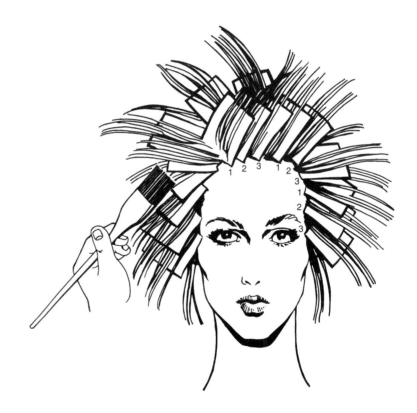

Figure 11-1

Use 3 formulas for a dimensional effect that creates movement:

1. **medium lift light blond**

2. **one darker golden blonde**

3. **one darker than client's color.**

Remember the Rules of Haircoloring, especially #4. Include enough of the darker tint formula to "ground" the hair color and give it a balanced effect. The beauty of planning your pattern is that it allows you creativity and helps customize your techniques.

1. *Prepare* foils (should be done before your scheduled appointment time).

2. *Prepare* your client for a tint, remembering to use tint apron or smock and gloves for yourself.

3. *Divide* the hair into the desired sections. Your vertical panels should be no wider than three inches.

4. Two choices:

   a. When making your **subsections**, begin parting at the bottom of each panel and work up to avoid slippage of the woven strands.

   b. If beginning at the top, lay your foil against the top of the head and push each strand up against it to avoid slippage.

5. When performing a weave procedure, *mix* very small amounts of product, enabling continuity in lift and timing. If bleach is used for the procedure, *stagger* volumes to control the lift. *Example:* first panel, use 10 volume, second use 20, etc.

6. Beginning in the area that requires the most lift *or* deposit effect, *part* a 1/4-inch subsection horizontally and *hold* at a 90° angle from the base with tension.

7. Holding a wiretail comb **parallel** to the section, beginning on the right side of the section, *insert* the wiretail comb with an up and down motion, weaving across subsection hair to the opposite side of the section (Figure 11-2).

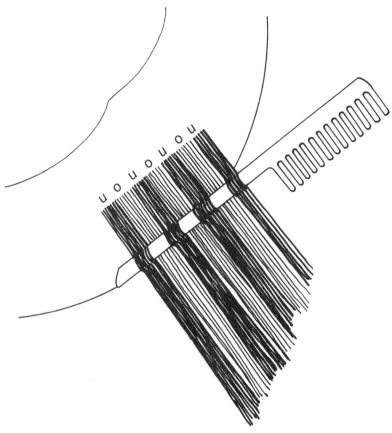

Figure 11-2

8. With the woven hair grasped in your thumb and forefinger, *push* the lower part of the subsection downward with the wiretail, separating the strands.

9. If using choice (a), take one piece of precut foil, *fold* the top 1/4 inch over the edge of the wiretail comb, making a clean, straight fold.

 **It's a toss up. Some people prefer the folded edge on the under side of the foil, some prefer the folded edge on the upper side.**

10. *Lift* the separated subsection and place the wiretail with foil attached directly under the parting against the scalp.

11. *Hold* the edges of foil from above, just past the edges of the subsectioned strands. *Slide* the wiretail comb out without disturbing the hair.

12. Still holding the thumb and finger against the foil, *load* the tint brush with your premixed formula. Starting 1/16 inch from the edge of foil, *apply* to all strands on foil with a downward motion, allowing for complete coverage and keeping the hair in place on the foil.

13. With your thumb and finger against the foil, *fold* the foil toward the scalp in half (Figure 11-3a); *fold* left side over to the center, then the right side *or* use the wiretail to crease the foil and bend it where desired (Figure 11-3b).

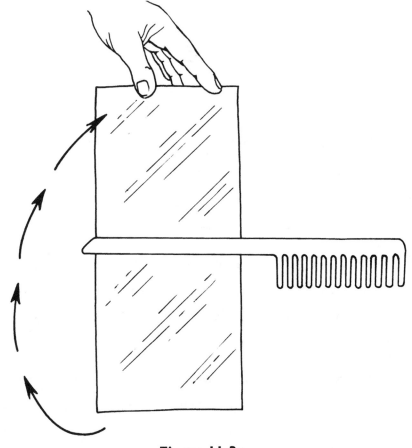

Figure 11-3a

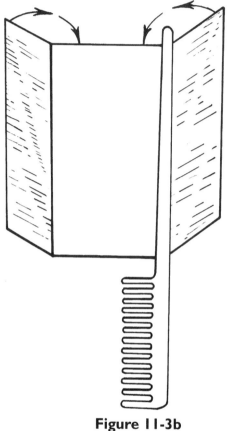

Figure 11-3b

14. For a heavy foiled effect, weave from each subsection. For more subtle results, apply to every other section.

15. More than one color may be used. Remember to frequently mix small batches of color, ensuring the proper processing.

16. When checking the processing, make sure to keep foils close to the scalp. If the first sections need removing before the last sections are complete, use a towel and water spray to stop processing action. Or use an **antioxidant** (product that halts oxidation).

17. Foils need not be removed individually when rinsing. Place the client's head in the shampoo bowl, *apply* medium temperature and water pressure, and foils will "rinse" from the hair.

18. *Shampoo* with the appropriate shampoo and conditioner.

19. *Style* to desired finish.

If you use choice (b), just *place* the straight edge of the foil against the section line at scalp and bend hair strand over it to hold the foil in place as you apply the product (Figure 11-4a). Then simply *fold* the edge back to the part so the foil bends in half to the scalp (Figure 11-4b).

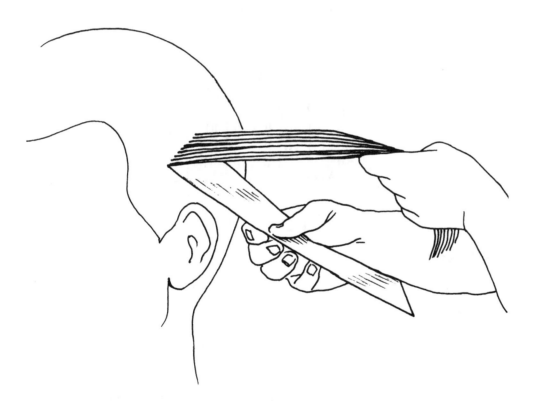

Figure 11-4a

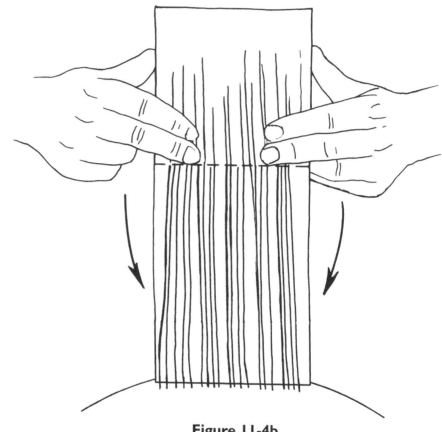

Figure 11-4b

Foil Procedure

The foil procedure would follow the same steps as the weave procedure, except for the following:

1. Rather than weaving pieces from each section, the horizontal subsection taken is much smaller, up to 1/16 inch depending on hair density. Color is then applied to the entire subsection, eliminating the weave process.

2. Color is applied to small sections mentioned in #1, but the uncolored subsections will be taken in 1/8- to 1/2-inch partings.

3. You may use one, two, three, or four colors and may also use bleach or a blonding creme mixture.

Standard Hair Coloring Activities Book

4. Processing, checking, and removal are identical to the weave procedure.

5. Due to the elimination of the weaving process, the foil technique enables the service to be completed more quickly. However, to ensure correct results extreme care must be taken to maintain very small subsections while applying.

As with any other technical service, practice builds speed. So practice, practice, practice!

LIGHTENER APPLICATIONS

Although this text is devoted to Level System color, a good **hair lightener** application is a bottle or brush application depending on the service given. On the scalp, bleaches are usually applied with the bottle to avoid any irritations.

Remember:

1. Don't follow in the part with your thumb or rub bleach into the scalp.

2. Don't comb hair with bleach product on the hair.

3. Don't **soap cap**.

4. *Never* apply heat onto the scalp bleach!

Virgin Lightener

Same as method L tint application.

Lightener Retouch Application

Same as tint retouch application except do not comb through or soap cap, and apply to new growth only.

Proper Removal of Bleach

1. Rinse product from hair with tepid to cool water.

2. Apply conditioning shampoo and shampoo gently but thoroughly.

3. Rinse with tepid to cool water.

4. Apply second shampoo and rinse.

 **If bleach is not thoroughly removed from hair, bleaching action will continue, causing severe damage and possible breakage.**

5. Condition hair and proceed with styling.

IIII➡ **ACTIVITY #1:** Foils and Weaves

OBJECTIVE: Gain skill with foil and weave techniques.

Materials:

- Aluminum foils cut to desired lengths, normally 4 to 6 inches wide by 4 to 8 inches long

- Tint bowls and brushes for each participant

- Conditioner to practice, if just learning

- Two duck bill clips and a wire tail comb for each student

- Optional: manikin heads to practice, or pair off and work on one another

Instructions:

1. Determine color formula to be used by each person.

2. Using the procedures outlined, do one half of the head using the foil technique and one half of the head using the weave technique. If students are practicing on one another, only one technique should be used.

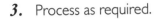

3. Process as required.

4. Remove foils, shampoo, rinse, and dry.

5. Check results.

Because foiling and weaving are such popular services in today's salon, students should practice as often as possible. Once skill is developed, substitute high lift tint or bleaching formulas for the practice session. Be careful! Always perform weaves and foils with an instructor's assistance!

IIII➡**ACTIVITY #2:** Color Applications

OBJECTIVE: Practice color applications.

Materials:

- Tint brushes, bowls, and bottles depending on application technique desired

- Formulations desired

- Tint capes

- Aprons

- Towels

- Comb

Instructions:

1. Using procedures outlined, apply color to 1/4 head subsections following each of these procedures:

   a. Brush application: retouch

   b. Bottle application: retouch

   c. Brush application: virgin lightener

   d. Bottle application: virgin lightener

2. Survey class preference from each application technique.

QUIZ

Match the simple steps from Method D and L.

Method D	Method L
_____	_____
_____	_____
_____	_____
	_____

a. Used to lighten hair one level or more.

b. Apply to regrowth using 1/8-inch partings.

c. Using 1/8-inch partings, apply fresh mixture to scalp and to the ends depending on the extent of porosity at the ends.

d. Immediately apply to shaft and ends, using 1/4-inch partings.

e. Process until shaft is almost exactly desired color.

f. Used to darken hair or lighten less than one level.

g. When scalp area is same color level as shaft and ends, remove color.

h. When processing is complete, shampoo.

i. Using 1/4-inch partings, apply starting 1/4 inch to 1/2 inch from scalp to porous ends.

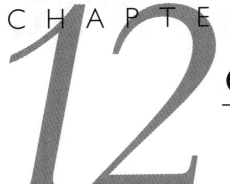

C H A P T E R

12

Coloring Techniques

In This Chapter You Will Learn:

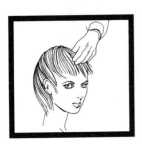

- **Procedures for coloring techniques:**
    Caramel-flaging
    Chunking
    TNT
    Marbleizing
    Flames
    Glazing, Glossing
    Angel-facing
    Bilevel color
    Corkscrew color
    Cocktail shampoo
    Twisters
    Multiples

Utilizing the information included so far in this manual, you would have a strong start on how to make a ton of money coloring hair if you were to stop right now. However, you will probably want to try to cover all the bases. **Technique** addresses method, expertise, and style. Your own technique for each type of color you do will definitely vary from others. Try as many as you can and practice selling these techniques to clinic clients. Invent new techniques of your own—have fun with it!

ADDITIONAL TECHNIQUES

Caramel-Flaging

Caramel-flaging produces brilliant highlights, lowlights, and shine on gray hair with a diffused regrowth line and low maintenance.

1. Divide hair in three sections. Then divide sections ear to ear (Figure 12-1).

optional

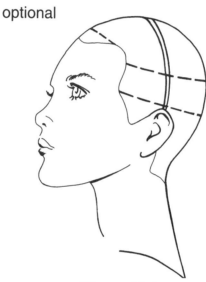

Figure 12-1

2. On 30% to 75% gray hair use three formulas:

    a. Formula #1 is two to four levels lighter than natural base color with 30 or 40 volume developer. May use high lift color, or lightening formula such as Blazing Hair.™

    b. Formula #2 is at the same level or one level lighter as the base color in golden or red-brown tone with 20 volume developer.

    c. Formula #3 is at the same level as the base color or one level darker in a natural tone with 10 or 20 volume developer.

On 75% to 100% gray hair, use only two formulas. The first formula is two to four levels lighter, your choice of warm or cool tones depending on the client's skin tones, with 20-30 volume developer. The second formula is the same level as the client's base color in a natural tone with 20 volume developer.

3. Using tiny slices (1/6 inch) and the foiling technique, apply color to all the hair.

4. On the top third of the head, apply Formula #1 alternating with Formula #2 and #3. Example: #1, #2, #1, #3, #1, #2, #1, #3—so there are more of #1 (Figure 12-2).

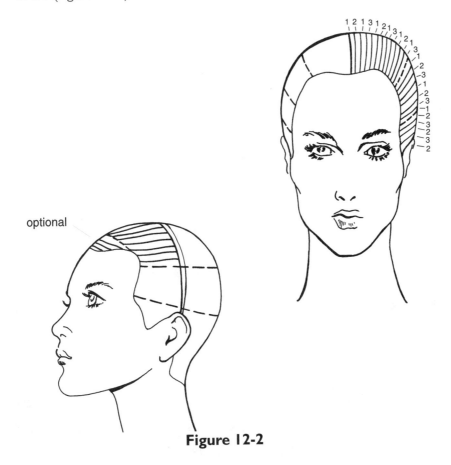

Figure 12-2

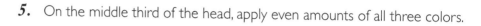

5. On the middle third of the head, apply even amounts of all three colors.

6. On the lower third of the head, apply Formula #3 alternating with #2. Use #1 with the first alternation only. Use #2 (base color) at all hairline areas and scalp to ensure 100% coverage.

 ▶ **This allows for a gradual darkening toward the base or foundation of the style and a diffused gray regrowth.**

7. Process 10 to 20 minutes until desired tones are achieved.

8. Remove foils; shampoo and condition.

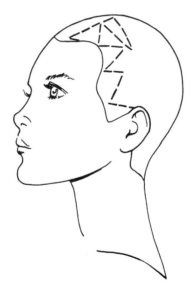

Figure 12-3

Chunking

Chunking gives dramatic highlights and accents to any style.

1. Create sections as follows:

   a. One-length hair: From top area along part and around facial area, divide large strands (up to 2 inches) into sections using diagonal partings or triangular shaped sections (Figure 12-3).

b. Layered hair: Do three layers of chunking. Part from ear to ear 1 1/2 inches from the base of the hairline.

2. Apply protective barrier creme or conditioner around parting with tint brush to avoid any seepage of lightener.

3. Lay large foil or plastic wrap at base of section.

4. Using 1/8-inch partings, apply lightener formula to all hair in each section (Figure 12-4).

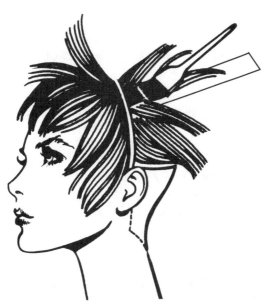

Figure 12-4

5. Fold foils up horizontally in half, then fold edges in to prevent seepage.

6. Continue with remainder of sections.

7. Process until desired highlight is achieved.

Although you might normally use dryer heat to process a foiled effect, this application goes right to the scalp, and might therefore cause severe irritation if heat is applied.

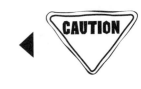

8. Remove foils; rinse, shampoo, and condition.

As an option for chunking, you might choose to apply a toning color over your chunking such as apricot or platinum to create drama and brightness!

Pinwheeling

Pinwheeling provides a kaleidoscope of color lights that illuminate a style from interior to perimeter.

1. Using alternating gold and red lifting formulas with 20 to 30 volume, brush tint onto the tips of a vent brush.

2. Following natural growth and the style lines of the cut, pull the vent brush into the style.

3. Alternate brushing with dotting the vent brush straight into hair, working around the head in a "wagon wheel" effect.

4. Process as recommended by the manufacturer.

5. Rinse, shampoo, condition, and style.

Tone on Tone

Tone on Tone (TNT) makes gorgeous corresponding tones that radiate shine—a very versatile technique! This process is great for gray coverage, makeovers, and tint-backs.

1. Apply desired tint to hair.

2. Mix a lightener application (only half the amount of normal formula is required).

3. After tint has processed 15 minutes, apply lightener as indicated.

4. Two options:

a. Using foils, weave out sections beginning at the temples in front and occipital in back, apply lightener formula directly over tint on hair.

Standard Hair Coloring Activities Book

b. Using pointed end of tint brush, select narrow partings. Apply lightener formula directly to random narrow sections of hair.

5. Process 10 to 20 minutes until desired effect is achieved.

For added tone on tone variety, apply lightener formula again after 5 minutes. Produces deep, light, and lighter effects all with the same tonal value.

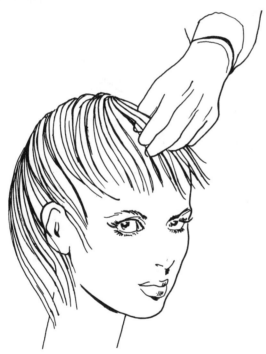

Figure 12-5

Marbleizing

Marbleizing combines ease of application with natural blends to create beautiful tones and bright lights. It creates a marblized, natural look.

1. Mix mild bleach formula (use 10 volume) in a tint bottle.

2. Put on gloves! Squeeze lightener onto your gloved hand.

3. Avoiding scalp, randomly squeeze lightener into hair (Figure 12-5).

4. Process 10 to 20 minutes without heat to desired lightness.

5. Two options:

    a. Remove bleach when processed, towel blot, then apply a deposit-only color with low volume developer. Process until color is intense and highlights are toned.

    b. Apply desired deposit formula over the bleach formula and process 10 to 20 minutes.

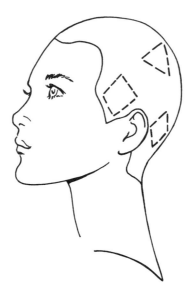

Figure 12-6

Flames

Flames create brilliant accents in gem colors. Although you might like several, the visual impact is strongest and most bold with just one.

1. Flames are best over a solid color. It can be bright red, orange or blue over black, or platinum. The trick is to make sure the flame is in bright contrast to the base color.

2. Select one triangular- or diamond-shaped section of hair on side, back, or top of head (Figure 12-6).

3. Prelighten to yellow for red or orange flames, to palest yellow for blue flames.

4. Rinse, shampoo, and dry.

5. Apply intense deposit-only color or toner to the prelightened section only.

6. Process until vibrant tone is reached.

7. Rinse, shampoo, condition, and style.

Glazing

Glazing generates a hint of highlight with no regrowth.

1. In applicator bottle combine 3–oz water with 3–oz desired highlight (red, gold, burgundy).

2. Apply at shampoo bowl.

3. Process for 5 minutes for shine and some highlighting or leave longer for more depth and drama.

Glossing

Glossing is similar to glazing, with brighter highlights and longer-lasting shine.

1. In applicator bottle combine 2–oz desired highlight (red, gold, burgundy) with 2–oz 10 volume developer and 2–oz protein conditioner.

2. Using 1/4-inch sections, quickly apply from scalp to ends.

3. Process for 5 to 20 minutes.

4. Rinse, shampoo, condition, and style.

Angel-facing

Angel-facing frames the face with dramatic blonde accents.

1. Select blonde tone desired.

2. Divide a 1 inch zigzag "halo" section on front hairline from the rest of the hair.

3. Secure remaining hair at back with clips. Apply protective barrier creme or conditioner around parting with tint brush to avoid any seepage of lightener.

4. Apply an on-the-scalp bleach formula as in a virgin lightener application to the front "halo" section. Use foil or plastic wrap to avoid contact with the remaining hair or skin.

5. Process until desired degree of lightness is achieved.

6. Rinse, shampoo, and condition.

7. Apply toner if needed.

8. Style.

Bilevel Coloring

Bilevel coloring is a favorite for accenting great haircut lines, making the hair look sculptured, thicker, and customized. Two different levels of color are used. Although it is not mandatory for them to be the same tonal group, they should be compatible, not conflicting.

1. Divide the hair into four equal sections, forehead to nape and ear to ear across the crest of the head. Make a parting from the temple at the front hairline back to just above the occipital bone at the back of the head (Figure 12-7). There are now eight subsections on the head. Clip sections in place.

2. Formula #1: The upper section will be two levels lighter than the natural base color with 20 volume developer. May use any color desired, but gold tones are usually preferred for this effect.

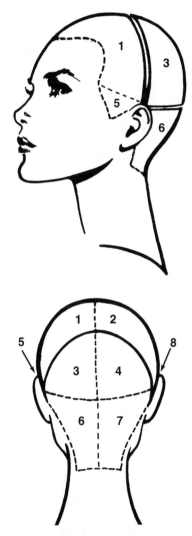

Figure 12-7

3. Formula #2: The lower section will be the same or one level darker than the natural base color and will use either 20 or 10 volume developer. This formula will naturally appear less gold due to its deeper color. You might also want to combine a natural tone with some ash tone to cut some of the warmth for this one.

4. Mix Formula #1 and apply the lighter Formula #1 to the upper four sections (1–4).

5. Mix Formula #2 and apply to lower four sections (5–8).

6. Allow the formulas to process 25 to 40 minutes depending on the manufacturer's instructions. Five minutes before the processing time is complete, use a tint comb to blend the lower section up into the upper section to avoid a **line of demarcation**. Comb up from bottom and out with a rolling motion to scoop the color from below into the upper.

7. After processing, rinse, shampoo, and recondition.

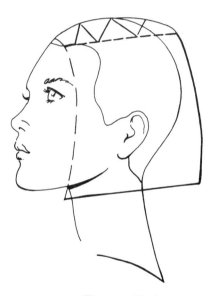

Figure 12-8

Twisters

Twisters create rippling highlights on one-length or bobbed hair. Use gold, red, burgundy, high lift blonde, or bleach.

1. From the top natural or planned part of the hair, separate a 1-inch section parallel to the part or the lower line of the cut.

2. Divide into triangular sections (Figure 12-8).

3. Each section is twisted from scalp to end, then clipped to prevent unraveling.

4. Lay foil or plastic wrap under twisted pieces, clip in place to stabilize.

5. Apply selected highlighting formula on top side only.

6. If using dryer heat, place another foil or wrap over sections and fold edges to secure.

7. Process for required time.

8. Rinse, shampoo, condition, and style.

Multiples

Multiples reflect multiple highlights while giving dimension and movement to any style. This technique is in common use in most salons on a daily basis.

1. Select three or four highlighting and lowlighting tones. *Example:* From a level 6 base—1-light golden blonde, 2-level 8 red-gold, 3-level 6 red, 4-level 4 natural brown.

2. Using weaving or foiling techniques, or combining both, alternate chosen colors. Use the highlighting colors the most on the top third of the head, then begin to use more of the level 6 and level 4 in the mid to lower sections.

3. Due to the number of colors being used, leave maximum 1/8 to 1/4 inch of natural color in between foiled or woven sections.

4. Process until desired color is achieved.

5. Rinse, shampoo, condition, and style.

Corkscrew Color

Corkscrew color radiates spirals of one or more highlights following the natural growth pattern in the hair.

1. Divide top, mid, and lower thirds of head in circular sections and clip.

2. Depending on natural flow of hair from crown and where hair is parted, plan a downward spiral pattern flowing from one section to the following section.

3. Pattern begins in crown and should end by crossing from either ear to opposite corner of nape.

4. Reversing your planned pattern, beginning in lower nape, draw an upward spiral to the top of the lowest section with the tail of a tint brush (Figure12-9).

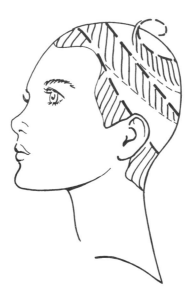

Figure 12-9

5. Apply desired highlighting color(s) such as red, gold, or burgundy to the hair in sweeping motions from part line to ends. This will cause radiating highlights from within your spiral.

6. Repeat upward spiral in middle section, then upper section. Top section requires less color and should "funnel" into crown cowlick (Figure 12-10).

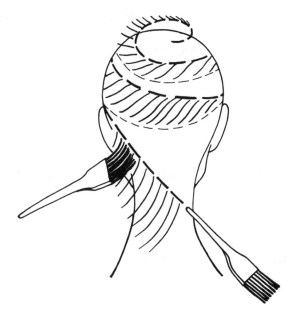

Figure 12-10

7. Process until desired highlights are achieved.

8. Rinse, shampoo, condition, and style.

Cocktail Shampoo

Cocktail shampoo makes for a more lasting effect similar to glossing.

1. Using any highlighting color desired, mix color formula using equal parts with 20 volume developer and conditioning shampoo.

2. Leave on for 5 to 25 minutes for a slight to more drastic effect.

Reverse Frost

Reverse frost (corrective color) is used for hair that is overlightened or for the client wishing a change.

Two methods of application are possible: Either pull strands to be darkened through a frosting cap or use the foil method. The amounts pulled or foiled depend on desired effect.

1. Apply combinations of desired colors for more variety and natural effect.

   Suggestions: beige blonde, light brown, light strawberry blonde, golden light brown.

2. Remember whenever you go two or more levels darker, a filler is often required.

3. Or use a color filler to enhance and add different highlights to select strands.

IIII➤**ACTIVITY #1:** Coloring Techniques Lotto

OBJECTIVE: Practice, practice, practice!

Instructions:

1. Write the different color techniques from this chapter on small pieces of paper.

2. Each student should draw one and perform in class on manikin or other student.

IIII➤**ACTIVITY #2:** Applied Techniques

OBJECTIVE: Familiarize students with the various coloring techniques.

Instructions:

1. Each student selects one technique.

2. Practice technique.

3. Recommend to clinic client.

4. Report results.

QUIZ

1. Outline procedure for TNT.

2. Write out the simple glazing formula.

3. Describe glossing.

4. What is bilevel coloring?

5. Describe marbleizing.

13

Helpful Hints

In This Chapter You Will Learn:

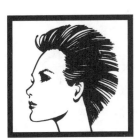

- **Review**

- **Helpful tips**

- **Reminders**

- **Business builders**

GENERAL TIPS

The best advice that can be offered is to *THINK FIRST!*

Tips to remember when coloring hair:

1. For best results use the H_2O_2 formulated by each color company as compatible for their own individual color lines.

2. Work with clean hair. Use clarifying shampoo before your color service.

3. Protect your client's skin at all times! Use a protective cream or petroleum jelly.

4. Do not use hair color on eyelashes or brows; it could cause blindness.

5. Do not use any color if scalp has sores or abrasions.

6. Color will not lift color!

7. If you're using a lifting formula on previously tinted hair, first use a color removal formula.

8. Almost always use your target level.

9. It is not possible to lift higher than level 10 with a tint.

10. The higher the volume of H_2O_2 you use, the more control you lose.

11. Are you lifting and drabbing or are you enhancing?

12. When lifting and drabbing, never use your target color.

13. All virgin hair is some shade of brown.

14. Remember, we don't deal with brown hair, even though all hair is brown; we deal with orange, red, yellow, etc.

15. Healthy hair pulls warm.

16. Porous hair pulls ash.

17. If going two or more levels darker, use filler.

18. You may need fillers with both deposit and high lift clients.

19. When doing a two-process color, lift half to one full level lighter than your target level to ensure desired results.

20. If in doubt, do a **strand test**.

21. Always do a patch test on a first-time color customer.

22. Never put color clients (especially on-the-scalp bleaches) under the dryer unless specifically endorsed by the manufacturer!

23. Plan your formula using many questions and answers in your consultation.

24. Have the product you need, and know when to mix it. As a general rule, when you are depositing only, you may mix all your product at once before applying any. When you are lifting and depositing, you might need to mix several small amounts to keep the lifting power consistent. Refer to the diagram showing lift and deposit cycles on page 48.

25. Wear gloves when you apply tint.

26. Have all your tools ready and organized for a quick, efficient application.

27. Proper application is essential for uniform coverage and end results. Apply quickly and thoroughly!

28. Write down all pertinent information on your client card.

29. Protect client from all possible leaks, stains, etc. (Use whatever method you usually use to protect neck and collars, as well as cream around hairline if client has sensitive skin or if you are using a dark color.)

30. Use enough product, but do not waste.

31. Neat, small, accurate applications make for successful coverage, and, contrary to what some might think, actually take less time and allow more control.

32. Anytime you add equal amounts of liquid to peroxide, the volume is approximately half (working volume).

33. Extra peroxide or a 2:1 ratio increases lifting ability of any volume.

34. Eighty percent of problems in tinting come from misjudging the base or existing level!

35. Usually, to make a missing level, use two parts of the lighter level color to one part of the darker level color. (Pigment weights average out.)

36. As a general rule of thumb for gray coverage, use the same amount of natural series as the percentage of gray in the hair.

37. For extremely resistant gray hair, use an ammonia booster product and 20 volume or a mild stripping shampoo before your color formula. This formula should be removed before applying the color formula. Some pre-softening formulas do not require removing before the color is applied.

38. Discard all mixed product not used.

39. Don't panic!

40. Remember that the Law of Color is universal.

41. Remember that any color can be fixed!

TIPS FOR BUILDING YOUR COLOR BUSINESS

1. Cross sell. Stylists should recommend that great haircuts can be enhanced with color.

2. Establish salon sales and techniques. If there aren't any recognized, consistent procedures and techniques, try to pioneer the idea with your coworkers.

3. Promote a color department within your salon! Sell the client in your chair on color and your coworkers. The visual results and word of mouth are the best advertising!

4. Listen closely for any openings clients give you to introduce them to color. (*Example:* The client mentions her hair is too dry, gray, or light after a perm, or she mentions her sister just got the most beautiful red color at her salon. This is the time to mention and sell some color!)

5. Recommend color. Start conversations that make your clients aware of all services available.

6. Wear a color look yourself. If you want to sell it, you have to wear it! You should change periodically with the tones of the season. *Example:* Great colors for fall are ambers, bronzes, golds, and topazes. You can be a walking advertisement for your salon and for your own techniques. A fashionable hairdresser attracts a fashionable clientele!

7. Keep thorough client files!

8. Education is essential! Use every opportunity to learn, update, get ideas, and find out what's happening in the industry!

9. Use videotape for practice consultation sessions, applications, and techniques. It's a great way to check up on yourself. Evaluate your performance, and target areas needing improvement. This will help you become more consistent, build your confidence, and develop communication skills.

10. Listen to client's problems and concerns.

11. Never leave the client alone in a room; never ignore your client.

12. Service plus attention to details means profits.

13. Stay out of ruts. Try a fresh approach occasionally, and suggest new looks frequently.

14. It is important to establish the credibility of professional hair color in your salon by using only professional products that are not available over the counter.

15. Whatever salon you work in, ask to see the color manual(s) and familiarize yourself with the ins and outs of the color product(s) your salon is using as soon as you begin working there.

16. Become familiar with the levels and tonal values of the color you will use. Practice recognizing the different colors and gain the confidence to accurately make color selections.

17. Experiment with hair swatches saved from your haircuts to actually see the superb results you can achieve with practice!

18. Attend as many color seminars and workshops as possible.

19. Let your satisfied clients advertise for you. When you do an outstanding color, send your business cards with that client. Tell her or him, "I know people are going to ask who did this great look on you, so please just hand these out when they do."

20. Remember to always recommend professional products for at-home maintenance of hair color, perms, or anything!

IIII➡**ACTIVITY #1:** Group Effort

OBJECTIVE: To brainstorm and increase sales.

Instructions:

1. Students form groups of four or five.

2. Each group develops one idea to promote color to clinic clients.

3. Each member of group performs plan daily.

4. Chart results daily using a chart such as Figure 13-1.

5. Report results monthly.

Group Plan:	Week #1	Week #2	Week #3	Week #4	
					TOTALS
Suggested:					
Performed:					
Group Plan:	Week #5	Week #6	Week #7	Week #8	
					TOTALS
Suggested:					
Performed:					

Figure 13-1 Use this chart to work with your student group.

||||➡**ACTIVITY #2:** Practical Application

OBJECTIVE: Encourage practice and develop ease of promoting colors.

Each student's assignment is to:

1. Research the best shampoos, conditioners, and styling aids for colored hair.

2. Practice recommending those products when giving color services in school clinic.

3. Record retail sales, and keep record for class using format found in Figure 13-2.

4. Report results.

Recommended Products (RP):	Shampoo	Conditioner	Clarifiers	Gels, Styling Aids	Hair Sprays, Pomades	Other	Total Recommended Products
Week #1 (W-1)							
Products Sold (PS):	Shampoo	Conditioner	Clarifiers	Gels, Styling Aids	Hair Sprays, Pomades	Other	Total Products Sold
Week #1 (W-1)							
(RP:W-2)							
(PS:W-2)							
(RP:W-3)							
(PS:W-3)							
(RP:W-4)							
(PS:W-4)							

Figure 13-2 Record product recommendations and sales on chart.

QUIZ

1. Color will not lift _____ .

2. Always use your target _____ .

3. Always do a _____ _____ on first-time color clients.

4. If lifting and drabbing, never use _____ .

5. Neat, accurate applications make for successful _____ .

6. Don't _____ .

7. Remember the _____ ____ _____ —it's universal.

8. Service and attention to details means _____ .

C H A P T E R

14

Activities and Tests

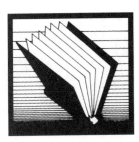

IIII▶ACTIVITY #1: Fill-in

OBJECTIVE: Practice.

orange-yellow (gold)	blue	orange
violet	red-orange	green
red	yellow	red-violet
blue-violet	blue-green	blue-yellow

Using the pool of words above:

1. List the primary colors.

_____

_____

_____

2. List the secondary colors.

_____

_____

_____

3. What are the tertiary colors?

_____   _____

_____   _____

_____   _____

Use the colors listed above to outline a color wheel.

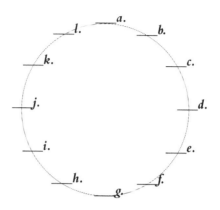

4. Complementary colors mixed together create brown. Pair the complementary colors.

_____&_____   _____&_____

_____&_____   _____&_____

_____&_____   _____&_____

||||► **ACTIVITY #2:** Fill-in

OBJECTIVE: More practice.

removing pigment (-) or lift   target

base   Level System

developer or hydrogen peroxide   adding pigment (+) or deposit

Shade System   oxidation

1. Measuring of light and dark _____

2. Coloring hair_____

3. Your starting color _____

4. Lightening hair _____

5. Desired color _____

6. H_2O_2 _____

7. Measuring by tonal value _____

8. Creates lift and deposit_____

IIII➡ ACTIVITY #3: Completion

OBJECTIVE: Practice.

a. What two things happen with oxidation?

_____

b. Which process refers to coloring hair or adding pigment?

_____

c. Which process refers to removing pigment?

_____

d. What is the client's main concern?

_____

e. What color is natural human hair?

_____

IIII➡ ACTIVITY #4: Matching

OBJECTIVE: Practice.

red/orange (R/O)   blue/violet (B/V)

yellow (Y)   orange/yellow (O/Y)

blue (B)   red (R)

violet/red (V/R)   violet (V)

pale yellow (PY)   orange (O)

Using the colors listed above, fill in the dominant remaining pigment in each level listed below:

1. Level 10 _____

2. Level 9 _____

3. Level 8 _____

4. Level 7 _____

5. Level 6 _____

6. Level 5 _____

7. Level 4 _____

8. Level 3 _____

9. Level 2 _____

10. Level 1 _____

⫸ ACTIVITY #5: Short Essay

Give an example of how you would use the chart in Activity #4:

_____

_____

_____

_____

_____

_____

⫸ ACTIVITY #6: Fill-in

To achieve an end result that is satisfactory to your client, you need to consider what three contributions: (Note answer 1 has two parts.)

1. _____

2. _____

3. _____

Standard Hair Coloring Activities Book

⫸ACTIVITY #7: Study Questions

1. What are the four basic components in permanent tint?

2. State the functions of each.

3. What two things do you consider when using a lifting (-) color?

4. What is aniline derivative?

5. What does a higher volume developer do?

6. What is DRP?

7. What color neutralizes the DRP at a level 8?

8. Level 7? 10? 6?

9. In Level System, what does the number for any given color in any given name line represent?

10. How about the letter?

11. Using general color information, what level and color base would you use to achieve each of the following?

	BASE	TARGET
a.	6N	8N
b.	5N	7N
c.	9N	6B
d.	10N	6N
e.	6N	8G (gold)
f.	8N	4N

For each of the above, decide if this process would be (-) or (+)

12. Define double-process blonding.

13. What does it mean when we say equal parts?

14. What is the formula for a bleaching or stripping shampoo?

15. What series is usually used to cover gray?

16. The three primaries mixed in unequal proportions equals?

17. What does working volume refer to?

18. What is pigment weight?

19. What two rules must you remember when you are drabbing and lifting?

20. Make a color wheel for each of the manufacturers in your school's inventory, then place each color where it should be according to the dominant color base for each series.

TEST #1

Name the three-part formula for success. (Note that answer 1 has two parts.)

1. _____

2. _____

3. _____

Fill in the steps for **Method D**:

1. _____

2. _____

3. _____

Fill in the steps for **Method L**:

1. _____

2. _____

3. _____

4. _____

Matching: Match each term with the best definition.

a. aniline derivative   *b.* ash   *c.* base color

d. certified hair colors   *e.* clarifier   *f.* cocktail shampoo

g. complementary color   *h.* corrective color   *i.* cortex

j. deposit   *k.* developer   *l.* dominant remaining pigment (DRP)

m. drab   *n.* equal parts   *o.* FDA

p. filler   *q.* foils   *r.* hair shaft

s. level   *t.* lift   *u.* metallic dyes

v. oxidative dyes   *w.* patch test   *x.* pH

y. porous   *z.* progressive tint   *aa.* retouch

bb. single process   *cc.* strand test   *dd.* target color

ee. tea effect   *ff.* warm zone   *gg.* weave

hh. working volume

1. The color that controls or overpowers other colors or hues within the lifting process of hair coloring. _____

2. The desired end result of color. _____

3. The use of aluminum strips or plastic to color small slices of hair. _____

4. This coal tar derivative creates the dye intermediates used in single-process permanent hair coloring. _____

5. The area of the hair shaft that develops tint more easily, within 1/2 inch of the scalp and body heat. _____

6. Hair with no warm tones. _____

7. A color application mixed with equal parts shampoo and developer that alters color less dramatically than permanent color. _____

8. Refers to the process of changing or correcting overlightened or damaged hair. Can also refer to major changes in the color of the hair. _____

9. A sample formula applied to a small portion of hair to check expected results. _____

10. Colorless intermediate molecules that develop into a color on mixing with hydrogen peroxide. _____

11. Your client's natural or existing hair color. _____

12. The diluted volume of hydrogen peroxide resulting after mixing the color portion of the formula. _____

13. The oxidizing agent, usually hydrogen peroxide, that causes the hair color formula to activate when mixed with color product. _____

14. Mixing of formula with same measures for each ingredient. _____

15. A skin test that determines sensitivity or allergy to a product or chemicals. In permanent hair coloring, any products containing aniline derivatives are required by the FDA to have such a test 24 hours prior to color services.

_____

16. A temporary replacement of lost pigment for overporous hair before the application of tint formula. _____

17. Describes condition of cuticle when it is raised and opened, allowing moisture and liquid to absorb. _____

18. Application of color formula to the new growth of the hair. _____

19. Tints (temporary) registered and deemed safe by the FDA. _____

20. Coloring technique using lighteners or deposit colors in which small amounts of hair are separated from subsections and tinted, then wrapped in foil or plastic to prevent leakage onto untinted hair. Currently the most popular and widespread method of off-the-scalp color. _____

21. Hair coloring procedure that lifts and deposits in one application. _____

22. A treatment that removes unwanted buildup on the hair. _____

23. Term used to describe the portion of each strand of hair that lies between 1/2 inch out from the scalp up to any porous ends. _____

24. Lightening of hair color due to high acidity of shampoos, rinses, or conditioners. Hair color is stripped from hair similar to the way tea lightens when lemon is added. _____

25. Colors that look best and brightest when placed next to each other. When mixed they neutralize one another. They are also opposite on the color wheel. _____

26. The portion of single-process oxidation when the color intermediates enter the cortex of the hair. _____

27. Refers to the degree of alkalinity or acidity of a solution. Neutral (water) is 7; anything below is acid; anything above is alkaline. _____

28. The main inner body (structure) of the hair shaft that is fibrous and contains the protein structure of the hair, as well as most of the natural color pigment of the hair. _____

29. Dyes that are made from metallic salts. They coat the hair and are progressive, getting increasingly dark and coated. They are extremely difficult to remove. Coloring over these dyes will create severe problems, such as breakage, melted hair, smoking hair, burns, etc. These dyes are not considered professional color treatments. _____

30. The exact measurement that determines the degree of light and dark in each color. Most color companies use 10 levels to determine their color formulas. _____

31. A term used to describe ash, cool, or blue tones that neutralize unwanted warm tones. Also used as a verb to describe the process of doing the same. _____

32. Any hair dye that continues processing until removed, or gets darker with each application. Level System colors are considered nonprogressive. _____

33. Food and Drug Administration _____

34. Removing, subtracting, or lightening color from the hair. Can also refer to the lightening ability of hair color or the amount a certain volume of developer will oxidize. _____

Fill-In

1. Always recommend a _____ treatment before a hair-color service.

2. _____ _____ is the reaction due to high acidity that strips red color from the hair.

3. Clients are _____ oriented.

4. The desired color is called _____ _____ .

5. An effective visual aid used during consultations is a _____ _____ .

TEST#2:

Color Wheel: List the colors.

Primary: _____

_____

_____

Secondary: _____

_____

_____

Tertiary: _____

_____

_____

_____

_____

_____

List the six complementary pairs.

_____

_____

_____

_____

_____

_____

Fill-in:

1. Name the darkest primary. _____

2. Name the brightest primary. _____

3. Name the lightest primary. _____

4. The three mixed in uneven amounts equal _____ .

5. When would you recommend a foil?

_____

6. When would you recommend a glazing?

_____

7. If a client wants to gradually go darker with hair that is too light, what would you recommend?

_____

Matching: Match each term with the best definition.

a. psychological	*b.* tint	*c.* texture
d. subsection	*e.* subtraction	*f.* synthetic pigment
g. temporary colors	*h.* tertiary	*i.* virgin hair
j. repigmentizing	*k.* result oriented	*l.* secondary
m. Shade System	*n.* primary	*o.* pigment
p. bleach	*q.* antioxidants	*r.* ammonia
s. alkaline substance	*t.* acid	*u.* oxidation
v. para-phenol pigment	*w.* coated hair	*x.* color base
y. color portfolio	*z.* pinwheeling	*aa.* multiporous
bb. metallic salts	*cc.* low lift	*dd.* line of demarcation
ee. consultation	*ff.* conditioning	*gg.* color removal formula
hh. dispensary	*ii.* end result	*jj.* hydrogen peroxide
kk. Law of Color		

1. Hair untreated by chemicals. _____

2. Word used to describe hair color or the process of coloring hair. Refers also to the tonal cast of the hair. _____

3. An ammonia gas solution in water; the most common source of alkaline substance in single- and double-process tint. Opens the cuticle to allow the color intermediates to penetrate. _____

4. Hair with a buildup of mineral, medications, styling products, conditioning waxes, etc. _____

5. An album of pictures or illustrations organized to display color choices in an attractive and effective manner. _____

6. The smaller divisions made within a section of hair, used for ultimate accuracy. _____

7. Colors made from acid dyes readily removed by shampooing. _____

8. Used in manufacturing, colors to help prevent the oxidation of the intermediates in the tube/canister. Increases shelf-life of product. _____

9. Treatments of cosmetic formulas that alter (improve) the state of the hair. _____

10. Mixture that removes excess pigment in the same manner as a stripping shampoo. _____

11. Involves the mental attitude of an individual. _____

12. Colors created when pairs of primaries are mixed: Y + R = O, R + B = V, B + Y = G. _____

13. The system of permanent haircoloring using shade or tonal values as its standard for categorizing. _____

14. A coal tar or aniline derivative most often found in haircolor and responsible for the pigmentation. _____

15. The matter that produces a specific color in hair or anything else. _____

16. In coloring, refers to the three basic colors of the color wheel that make up all other colors when combined in different variations with one another. _____

17. Having a pH below 7.0; any matter that produces or supplies hydrogen ions in solution. _____

18. Refers to the diameter of each shaft of hair. Usually categorized by fine, medium, or coarse. _____

19. Color that is not natural to the structure of the hair. Usually derived from para-phenol diamines. _____

20. Filler _____

21. An ingredient in hair color that has a pH greater than 7.0, causing the cuticle to open and permanent color to enter the cortex. _____

22. Product used to lighten hair, usually mixed with hydrogen peroxide and highly alkaline. _____

23. Occurs when permanent tints are mixed with hydrogen peroxide, causing lift and deposit of natural and synthetic pigments. _____

24. The line of regrowth between colored hair and natural, untinted (virgin) hair. _____

25. Lead, silver, iron, and bismuth, compounds created by combining a base and an acid. Used in some color products although not recommended by professionals. _____

26. Putting more emphasis on the finished effect than the process by which it is achieved. _____

27. Term used for lift or removal of pigment. _____

28. Color created when a primary is mixed with its neighboring secondary.
_____

29. Highlighting effect applied with a vent brush. _____

30. The portion of the hair color mixture that connects or holds the other ingredients together. Can be liquid, creme, shampoo, protein, etc. May also refer to the dominant color in any given shade or series. _____

31. Means maximum deposit, minimal lifting ability (less than one level). _____

32. Hair that has more than one porosity within the strand. _____

33. The process of discovering the client's desired end results. _____

34. The finished effect _____

35. The common oxidizing substance mixed with hair tint that develops the hair color and causes oxidation. _____

36. The elementary rules that form the foundation of all reference to color, including the primary colors and how they combine to make all other color. _____

37. The designated place in a salon or school where supplies are prepared, dispensed, or stored. _____

CHAPTER

15

Answers to Activities and Quizzes

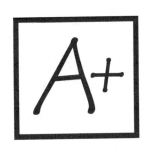

CHAPTER 1

Quiz: 1. The Level System is the numerical system of judging color in levels, or numbers, one level being a measure of light or dark in the hair. **2.** Color. **3.** The process of changing or correcting overlightened or damaged hair. Can also refer to major changes in the color of the hair. A technician will use corrective coloring when changing or correcting the color of the hair. Considered profitable because the corrective color process might involve several processes as well as much time, thereby making it more profitable. **4.** To cover or camouflage gray hair. **5.** It makes the hair appear thicker and makes a haircut appear sculptured.

CHAPTER 2

▐▐▐▶**Activity #1: 1)** b **2)** h **3)** f **4)** d **5)** e **6)** a **7)** c **8)** j **9)** i **10)** g

▐▐▐▶**Activity #2:** In any order; yellow and violet, blue and orange, red and green, yellow/orange (gold) and blue/violet, orange/red and blue/green, violet/red and green/yellow **1)** Y **2)** Y/O **3)** O **4)** O/R **5)** R **6)** V/R **7)** V **8)** B/V **9)** B **10)** B/G **11)** G **12)** G/Y

Quiz: 1) yellow, red, and blue **2)** orange, violet, and green **3)** brown **4)** Law of Color **5)** yellow and violet, blue and orange, red and green, yellow/orange and violet, orange/red and blue/green, violet/red and green/yellow

CHAPTER 3

IIII➡**Activity #1:** yellow and violet; red and green; and blue and orange

CHAPTER 4

IIII➡**Activity #2: A)** 3 **B)** 4 **C)** DRP not a factor **D)** 2 **E)** DRP not a factor

Special problems to consider are: for C-level 10 to level 3 natural requires a filler or repigmentation. If the hair is a level 10, most of the pigment necessary to achieve a *natural* level 3 is absent from the hair. Because all darker hair colors must have a dominance of blue pigment to make the color darker, the filler must have both red and yellow pigment to balance and make a natural effect. In this case, the correct fillers would be gold and deep red to balance the deep color pigment for a level 3. When depositing color, you usually use your target color, so you would use level 3 natural after filling.

Special problems to consider for E: level 8 to level 6 red also requires a filler or repigmentation. Because the desired target color in this formula is a 6 *red*, you need to guarantee there is adequate orange in the hair to make a nice, vibrant base for the level 6 red color you will use to achieve maximum deposit.

IIII➡**Activity #3: A)** subtraction **B)** subtraction **C)** addition **D)** subtraction **E)** addition

Quiz: **1)** temporary **2)** permanent **3)** deposit-only **4)** permanent **5)** permanent **6)** semipermanent

Quiz: 1) pigment and base **2)** pigment, base, and alkaline substance **3)** pigment, base, alkaline substance, and hydrogen peroxide

Standard Hair Coloring Activities Book

CHAPTER 5

Quiz: 1) pigment—responsible for tonal value, made of aniline derivative **2)** base—what holds the product together, can be creme, gel, oil, shampoo, etc. **3)** alkaline substance—usually ammonia, responsible for opening the cuticle and promoting lightening action **4)** hydrogen peroxide—responsible for lift and development of pigment—it is the hydrogen peroxide that causes oxidation

CHAPTER 6

Quiz: 1) client's beginning hair color, either natural or tinted **2)** desired result **3)** cool—green, blue, and violet; warm—red, orange, and yellow **4)** 0–30% **5)** 60–100% **6)** tea effect **7)** W, L, R, and blondes **8)** 1. Hair should be lighter on ends than at the base of the hairshaft; 2. Hair should be lighter on the surface than underneath; 3. Face-line hair should be lighter than the hair behind it; 4. The darker hair should always be the dominant color **9)** coating on hair, porosity, texture, previously tinted hair, percentage gray, tenacity, medications, chlorinated hair, and metallic dyes **10)** end result

CHAPTER 7

||||➡**Activity #3: a)** To achieve orange hair: with dark strands, simply prelighten with bleach and remove lightener when orange is visible. To achieve orange hair on mid- to light-colored swatches, you will have to apply an orange-based color, filler, or stain. **b)** To achieve yellow on darker strands, prelighten with bleach and remove lightener when yellow is visible. Yellow on light strands is more difficult to achieve, but can be done with temporary or semipermanent stains, or by dipping in diluted yellow food coloring. **c)** Brassy can be achieved on darker hair (level 3 and

up) by using a high lift tint with the highest volume developer (40), and removing after only half the processing time, or by prelightening with bleach and removing at the brassy yellow/orange stage. On black hair, brassy can be achieved by using bleach; remove at level 8 or brassy yellow/orange. Brassy can be achieved on light hair by applying a gold-based color formula or semipermanent color with gold intensifier. **d)** Silver/ash can be achieved through either prelightening or using extremely light hair, then applying a blue/violet based color at the highest level (10, 11, or 12 depending on different manufacturers). It can be exaggerated by applying blue-violet or silver concentrate. **e)** Violet or mauve is achieved by using violet-based color or toner on extremely pale yellow or white hair.

IIII➡ **Activity #4: a)** To neutralize orange, use blue-based color with 20 volume developer, preferably at the next lightest level to avoid making swatch look darker. **b)** To neutralize yellow, use a violet-based color or toner, usually with 10 or 5 volume developer. **c)** To neutralize brassy/gold effects, use blue/violet-based color with 20 volume developer. **d)** To neutralize silver/ash tones, apply a gold-based color at the same level, with 10 or 20 volume developer. You many also want to use a gold concentrate added to your formula. **e)** To neutralize violet or mauve, use a light gold-based color with 10 or 20 volume developer. Other options: For the silver/ash and violet or mauve colors you can apply the color removal formula described in Chapter 9. If you have sufficient swatches for experimentation, try the color solutions described above and the color removal formula, then compare results!

Quiz: 1) hair—base and target; color; and hydrogen peroxide **2)** hair **3)** opposite **4)** same **5)** peroxide

CHAPTER 8

Quiz: 1) repigmentation **2)** to ensure proper tonal depth of the color and to avoid fadage **3)** two or more levels darker, fadage problems, and tonal value is off **4)** two **5)** primary

CHAPTER 9

Quiz: 1) 2–oz H_2O_2, 2–oz powdered bleach, 1–oz shampoo, 1–oz conditioner **2)** the one that is right for your type of application: on the scalp, avoid powders **3)** yes, always **4)** frequent retouches **5)** Apply at the shampoo bowl, often on wet hair. Apply quickly and evenly with a tint brush and broad sweeps of the brush. Monitor the entire time the product is on the head, shampoo with conditioning shampoo, and recondition. **6)** oil, creme, and powder **7)** oil or creme **8)** powder

CHAPTER 10

▥➤**Activity #1: 1)** If using light swatches, you will need to fill with gold and orange, then use a level 6 natural to achieve the level 6N. Use 10 or 20 volume developer, and process until the desired color is achieved. **2)** On the light swatches, fill with gold/orange, then apply level 7 gold with 10 or 20 volume. Process until the desired color is achieved. **3)** On the light swatches, use gold and deep orange/red filler, then apply level 4 natural with 10 or 20 volume developer. Watch carefully—at this depth, the color will develop quickly. **4)** On the light swatches, use gold and deep orange/red filler, then apply level 4 red with 20 volume. You might like to try a small amount of red concentrate in your color formula. Process for as long as required to get the maximum red deposit.

Quiz: 1) 1. fix what others have done; 2. image change; 3. tint-backs; 4. color removal; 5. correcting off-colors **2)** fillers or repigmentizing, reconditioning **3)** Follow the manufacturer's advice, or go with a filler that has deep red plus gold for levels 1–5; orange for levels 6 and 7, and gold for levels 8–10. The intensity of the filler should be determined by the level of your target color. **4)** a. color removal treatment, b. reconditioning, c. filling **5)** Fill with gold, apply a level 8 natural with 10 or 20 volume developer. Process until desired color is achieved.

CHAPTER 11

Quiz: Method D: b, d, f, and h. **Method L:** a, i, e, c, and g

CHAPTER 12

Quiz: 1) TNT: 1. Apply desired tint to hair; 2. Mix a lightener application; 3. After tint has processed for 15 minutes, apply lightener with either foils or by randomly selecting pieces for application with pointed end of tint brush. Process 10–20 minutes until desired effect is achieved. **2)** In an applicator bottle combine 3–oz water with 3–oz desired highlight. Apply at shampoo bowl. Process for 5 minutes for shine and some highlighting, longer for more depth and drama. **3)** Glossing is similar to glazing, with brighter highlights and longer-lasting shine. **4)** Bilevel coloring accents haircut lines, makes hair look sculptured, thicker, and customized. Two different levels of color are used. **5)** Marbleizing combines ease of application with natural blends to create beautiful tones and bright lights.

CHAPTER 13

▶ **Activity #1:** Each group of students should have a chart that tracks: 1. the idea being promoted, 2. names of all participants, 3. daily results, 4. total results after 1 month

▶ **Activity #2:** Each student should have a chart that tracks: 1. the recommended shampoos, conditioners, and styling aids for colored hair, 2. daily recommendations, 3. total results after 1 month

Quiz: **1)** color **2)** level **3)** patch test **4)** target color **5)** coverage **6)** panic **7)** Law of Color **8)** profit

CHAPTER 14

▶ **Activity #1:** **1)** yellow, red, blue **2)** orange, violet, green **3)** yellow/orange (gold), orange/red, red/violet, blue/violet, blue/green, green/yellow **a.** yellow, **b.** gold or yellow/orange, **c.** orange, **d.** red/orange, **e.** red, **f.** red/violet, **g.** violet, **h.** blue/violet, **i.** blue, **j.** blue/green, **k.** green, **l.** green/yellow **4)** yellow/violet; orange/blue; red/green; gold/blue-violet; orange-red/blue-green; violet-red/green-yellow

▶ **Activity #2:** **1)** Level System **2)** adding pigment (+) or deposit **3)** base **4)** removing pigment (-) or lift **5)** target **6)** developer or hydrogen peroxide **7)** Shade System **8)** oxidation

▶ **Activity #3:** **a.** lift and deposit **b.** deposit **c.** lift **d.** end result **e.** brown

▶ **Activity #4:** **1)** PY **2)** Y **3)** O/Y **4)** O **5)** R/O **6)** R **7)** V/R **8)** V **9)** B/V **10)** B

▶ **Activity #5:** This chart is used when lifting or lightening color to determine the dominant remaining pigment at the target level. To achieve the desired end result, this chart helps you decide whether you will be using a color formula that enhances or drabs the DRP.

▐▐▐▶**Activity #6:** **1)** hair; base and target **2)** color **3)** H_2O_2

▐▐▐▶**Activity #7:** **1)** base, pigment, NH_3, and H_2O_2 **2)** Base is what holds the product together. It can be creme, gel, oil, shampoo, etc. Pigment is responsible for tonal value, made of aniline derivative. The alkaline substance is usually ammonia and is responsible for opening the cuticle and promoting lightening action. Hydrogen peroxide is responsible for the lift and development of pigment. Hydrogen peroxide causes oxidation. **3)** The DRP at target level and if you are enhancing or drabbing that color. **4)** A coal tar derivative that creates the dye intermediates used in single-process permanent hair coloring. **5)** Keeps the color formula lifting longer. **6)** dominant remaining pigment **7)** blue/violet **8)** blue; pale violet; blue/green **9)** The level or degree of light and dark in the hair. **10)** tonal value **11) a.** level 8 blue/violet base and developer to lift two levels (usually 30 volume), usually process 30–45 minutes, **b.** level 7 blue base and developer to lift two levels (usually 30 volume), usually process 30–45 minutes, **c.** fill with gold and orange, use a level 6 gold base and 10 or 20 volume developer, process 20–30 minutes, **d.** fill with gold and orange pigment. Use a level 6 natural with 10 volume, process for 20–30 minutes, **e.** level 8 natural to allow the gold DRP to be enhanced and developer to lift two levels (usually 30 volume), process for 30–45 minutes, **f.** fill with deep red pigment. Use level 4 natural and 10 volume, process for 20–30 minutes. **a.** (-) **b.** (-) **c.** (+) **d.** (+) **e.** (-) **f.** (+) **12)** Prelightening with bleach, then toning. **13)** Measurements in any formula that are identical. Example: 1–oz color and 1–oz developer. **14)** 2–oz H_2O_2, 2–3 scoops bleach, 1–oz shampoo, 1–oz conditioner **15)** N or natural **16)** brown **17)** the diluted strength of developer after being mixed with color, conditioners, etc. **18)** the amount of pigment concentration at each level of artificial hair color **19)** 1. Always use your target level or higher. 2. Never use your target color. **20)** For each instructor to review and correct.

ANSWERS TO TESTS

Test #1: 1) hair; base and target **2)** color **3)** H_2O_2 **Method D:** 1. Using 1/8-partings, apply to regrowth on entire head. 2. Immediately apply to the shaft and ends, using 1/4-partings. 3. When processing is complete, shampoo. **Method L:** 1. Using 1/4-inch partings, apply starting 1/4 to 1/2 inch from the scalp to porous ends. 2. Process until shaft is almost desired color. 3. Using 1/8-partings, apply fresh mixture to scalp area and ends depending on the porosity. 4. When scalp is same color level as shaft and ends, remove color.

Matching: 1) l **2)** dd **3)** q **4)** a **5)** ff **6)** b **7)** f **8)** h **9)** cc **10)** v **11)** c **12)** hh **13)** k **14)** n **15)** w **16)** p **17)** y **18)** aa **19)** d **20)** gg **21)** bb **22)** e **23)** r **24)** ee **25)** g **26)** j **27)** x **28)** i **29)** u **30)** s **31)** m **32)** z **33)** o **34)** t

Fill-in: 1) clarifier **2)** tea effect **3)** result **4)** target color **5)** color portfolio

Test #2: Primary: red, yellow, blue **Secondary:** orange, violet, green **Tertiary:** yellow/orange, orange/red, red/violet, blue/violet, blue/green, green/yellow **Complementary pairs:** yellow and violet; blue and orange; red and green; yellow/orange and blue/violet; orange/red and blue/green; red/violet and green/yellow

Fill-in: 1) blue **2)** red **3)** yellow **4)** brown **5)** when the client wants highlights, or multiple colors **6)** when the client wants a slightly brighter effect **7)** reverse frost using a filler first, and reconditioning until the tinted hair is the client's desired color, then gradually color more and more of the hair darker

Matching: 1) i 2) b 3) r 4) w 5) y 6) d 7) g 8) q 9) ff 10) gg 11) a 12) l 13) m 14) v 15) o 16) n 17) t 18) c 19) f 20) j 21) s 22) p 23) u 24) dd 25) bb 26) k 27) e 28) h 29) z 30) x 31) cc 32) aa 33) ee 34) ii 35) jj 36) kk 37) hh

C H A P T E R

16

Manufacturers' Hotline Numbers

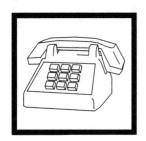

Listed below are all hotline numbers currently available for major manufacturers of hair color. Why not telephone and request all information available from each? By doing so you familiarize yourself with the ins and outs of each product, thereby increasing your ease and comfort level with hair color.

Aloxxi Chroma	1-805-968-6900
Aveda	1-800-283-3224
Clairol	1-800-221-4900
Colorly	1-800-621-4859
Dikson	1-416-298-2309 (phone collect)
Framesi	1-800-245-6323
Goldwell	1-800-333CHIC
Indola	1-800-333-0009
Joico	1-800-44JOICO
Logics (Clairol)	1-800-356-4427
L'Oréal	1-800-345-5012
Matrix (SOCOLOR)	1-800-282-2822
Redken	1-800-423-5280
Regal	1-800-REGAL 97
Renbow	1-800-352-3204
Revlon	1-800-223-2339
Schwarzkopf	1-800-433-5980
Scruples	1-800-457-0016 or 1-888-727-8753
Sunglitz	1-800-237-9175
Tressa	1-800-879-8737
Wella	1-800-THE-COLOR

Glossary

A

acid—Having a pH below 7.0; any matter that produces or supplies hydrogen ions in solution.

alkaline substance—An ingredient in hair color that has a pH greater than 7, causing the cuticle to open and permanent color to enter the cortex.

ammonia (NH_3)—An ammonia gas solution in water; the most common source of alkaline substance in single- and double-process tint. Ammonia opens the cuticle to allow the color intermediates to penetrate. When mixed with hydrogen peroxide, it activates the oxygen to create oxidation.

angel-facing—Lightening technique that creates a halo effect around the face with dramatic blonde accents.

aniline derivative—A coal tar derivative that creates the dye intermediates used in single-process permanent haircoloring.

antioxidants— Used in manufacturing colors to help prevent the oxidation of the intermediates in the tube/canister; increases shelf-life of product.

application—Method of applying color to the hair.

ash—Hair with no warm tones

B

base—Ingredient of permanent haircolor that holds the product together; can be a creme, oil, protein, wax, gel, or shampoo.

base color (BC)—Your client's natural or existing hair color

bilevel coloring—Coloring technique using two different level formulas to give haircuts a sculptured, thicker, and more customized effect.

bleach—Product used to lighten hair. Usually mixed with hydrogen peroxide and highly alkaline.

blend—To combine areas of application after processing (shaft to ends, dimensional light to dark) to ensure proper consistency in color results.

brassy—Term used to describe color that is off-color and contains too much warmth, either gold or orange.

buffer—Substance or mixture that resists changes of pH.

C

caramel-flaging—Gray coverage created by using three formulas of tint that produce highlights, lowlights, and shine with a diffused regrowth line and low maintenance.

certified hair colors—Tints (temporary) registered and deemed safe by the FDA.

chelating agents—Act to remove unwanted buildup, such as metallic ions and metallic deposits; common ingredient in cleansing or clarifying shampoos.

chunking—Highlighting effect producing dramatic lightened strips.

clarifier—A treatment that removes unwanted buildup on the hair.

cleansing shampoo—Shampoo or treatment that removes unwanted buildup containing chelating agents.

coated hair—Hair with a buildup of mineral, medications, styling products, conditioning waxes, etc.

cocktail shampoo—A color application mixed with equal parts shampoo and developer that alters color less dramatically than permanent color.

color base—The portion of the hair color mixture that connects or holds the other ingredients together. Can be liquid, cream, shampoo, protein, etc. May also refer to the dominant color in any given shade or series.

colorizing—Coloring technique that mixes equal parts color, 10 volume developer, and protein conditioner.

color portfolio—An album of pictures or illustrations organized to display color choices in an attractive and effective manner.

color refreshers—Temporary colors in the form of mousse

color removal formula—Mixture that removes excess pigment in the same manner as a stripping shampoo.

color wash—A coloring service used to highlight or brighten existing tones without drastic change to the base color.

color wheel—The universal guide for color mixing and formulation

complementary color—Colors that look best and brightest when placed next to each other. When mixed, they neutralize one another. They are also opposite on the color wheel.

composition—Construction, formation, configuration, or design of an element or article.

conditioning—Treatments of cosmetic formulas that alter (improve) the state of the hair.

consultation—The process of discovering the client's desired end results.

contouring—A method creating sculptured effects with the use of two or more tones.

cool—Lack of warmth, no warm tones; ash

corkscrew color—Tinting process that creates a spiral of highlights radiating from crown to nape.

corrective color—Refers to the process of changing or correcting overlightened or damaged hair; can also refer to major changes in the color of the hair.

cortex—The main inner body (structure) of the hair shaft that is fibrous and contains the protein structure of the hair, as well as most of the natural color pigment of the hair.

cosmetic effect—Results contributing to the creation or enhancement of physical attributes.

counterparts—Items that are similar, corresponding, complementary, or equal.

creme oil bleach—A bleach that contains oil, making it more gentle on the scalp.

cuticle—Extremely thin protective outer layer of the hair shaft consisting of overlapping scales. Condition of cuticle determines porosity of hair.

D

decolorize—The process of removing natural or artificial pigment from the hair.

demineralize—The process of removing mineral coatings from the hair.

deposit (+)—The portion of single-process oxidation when the color intermediates enter the cortex of the hair.

developer—The oxidizing agent, usually hydrogen peroxide, that causes the hair color formula to activate when mixed with color product.

dimensional effect—An effect that adds contoured, sculptured, or thickening effects with color.

direct dye—Used in semipermanent color, it is a molecule that has color.

discoloration—A shade that is unnatural or off-tone

dispensary—The designated place in a salon or school where supplies are prepared, dispensed, or stored.

dispersing agents—Matter that causes other ingredients within a solution or mixture to mix and spread completely.

dominance—Power, control, or command over something

dominant remaining pigment (DRP)—The color that controls or overpowers other colors or hues within the lifting process of haircoloring.

double-process—The process that includes first prelightening or decolorizing the hair with bleach or like substance, then coloring with an oxidation tint or toner.

drab—A term used to describe ash, cool, or blue tones that neutralize unwanted warm tones. Also used as a verb to describe the process of doing the same.

E

end result—The finished effect

enhance—To intensify, strengthen, or embellish something.

equal parts—Same measures for each ingredient when formulating.

F

fade—The loss of color intensity and depth

fear factor—Anxiety felt when attempting to perform a service.

filler—A temporary replacement of lost pigment for overporous hair before the application of tint formula.

flames—Dramatic color accents in the hair created by prelightening hair, then toning with vibrant accent colors.

foils—The use of aluminum strips or plastic to color small slices of hair.

Food and Drug Administration (FDA)—Federal agency that regulates materials used in haircoloring.

formulation—A mixture of two or more ingredients. In haircoloring it usually involves color plus H_2O_2.

G

glazing—Producing minimum regrowth by mixing tint with water.

glossing—Provides minimum coverage while producing brightness and shine.

gold bands—Undesirable brassy or gold tones that occur when hair is not lightened long enough.

H

hair lightener—Any product that helps to lighten the hair, such as bleach, blonding cremes, ammonia boosters, activators, etc.

hair shaft—Term used to describe the portion of each strand of hair that lies between 1/2 inch out from the scalp up to any porous ends.

henna—A vegetable dye that originated in Asia centuries ago. It is a progressive and coating dye.

highlighting—A process that creates a lighter color on selected strands to produce contrast and brighten the hair color.

humectants—A chemical or substance in hair products helping the hair to retain moisture (water).

hydrogen peroxide (H₂O₂)—The common oxidizing substance mixed with hair tint that develops the hair color and causes oxidation.

I

image—Client's fashion and life-style preferences

imbalance—Uneven or unmatched, not stable

insoluble—Will not mix with water.

intensified—Effects that are strengthened or emphasized.

intermediates—Colorless dye molecules that develop into permanent hair color when mixed with other intermediates during oxidation.

intermix—One color's ability to mix with others.

K

keratin—The strong, fibrous, insoluble protein that comprises approximately 95% of the hair shaft.

L

Law of Color—The elementary rules that form the foundation of all reference to color, including the primary colors and how they combine to make all other color.

level—The exact measurement that determines the degree of light or dark in each color. Most color companies use 10 levels to determine their color formulas.

Level System—The system of permanent haircoloring using levels of color as its standard.

lift (-)—Removing, subtracting, or lightening color from the hair. Can also refer to the lightening ability of hair color or the amount a certain volume of developer will oxidize.

light absorption—The ability of the hair to absorb light. Lighter hair reflects more; the darker the hair, the more light it absorbs.

light reflection—Hair's ability to reflect

lightening—The process of removing or subtracting pigment from the hair.

line of demarcation—The line of regrowth between colored hair and natural, untinted (virgin) hair.

low lift—Maximum deposit, minimal lifting ability (less than one level).

lowlighting—Adds depth by coloring certain strands or areas of hair darker; can create a highlighting effect by providing contrast.

M

marbleizing—Technique of application involving squeezing lightening formula on hair with hands, then depositing a highlighting color.

maximum lift—The maximum removal of pigment.

melanin—Natural pigment of the hair, most of which is usually found in the cortex.

metallic dyes—Dyes that are made from metallic salts. They coat the hair and are progressive, getting increasingly dark and coated. They are extremely difficult to remove. Coloring over these dyes will create severe problems, such as breakage, melted hair, smoking hair, burns, etc. These dyes are not considered professional color treatments.

metallic salts—Lead, silver, iron, and bismuth. Compounds created by combining a base and an acid. Used in some color products although not recommended by professionals.

molecules—Groups of atoms joined by chemical bonds.

multiples—Use of highlights and lowlights to create dimension and movement in a style.

multiporous—Hair that has more than one porosity within the strand.

N

natural—Organic, existing in nature, not artificial.

O

opposites—A reference to colors facing one another, diametric or contrasting, on the color wheel.

overlap—To apply or spread color over regrowth area onto previously colored hair, often causing a line of demarcation.

oxidation—A reaction occurring when permanent tints are mixed with hydrogen peroxide, causing lift and deposit of natural and synthetic color pigments. It has a limited effectiveness, usually determined by the volume of the H_2O_2 used, but can also be dictated by the percentage of NH_3 in a formula.

oxidative dyes—Colorless intermediate molecules that develop into a color on mixing with hydrogen peroxide.

P

parallel—Lines that run an equal distance from one another forever, never intersecting.

para-phenol pigments —A coal tar or aniline derivative most often found in hair color and responsible for the pigmentation.

para-phenylenediamine (PPD)—The basic, original aniline derivative used in single-process haircoloring.

part—In color formulations, it refers to dividing a whole amount into smaller measures. *Example:* 1 part = 1 oz color + 1 part = 1 oz developer. Makes 2 parts color formula, also referred to as equal parts. In hairstyling, part refers to the line created when dividing the hair into sections or subsections.

partings—Creating areas or sections by dividing the hair with a line or part and combing away from that line.

patch test—A skin test that determines sensitivity or allergy to a product or chemicals. In permanent haircoloring, any products containing aniline derivatives are required by the FDA to have such a test 24 hours prior to color service.

permanent hair color—Synthetic or organic dye that penetrates into the cortex of the hair and does not wash out.

pH—Refers to the degree of alkalinity or acidity of a solution. Neutral (water) is 7; anything below is acid; anything above is alkaline.

philosophy—Outlook, conviction, or viewpoint

pigment—The matter that produces a specific color in hair or anything else.

pigment weight—The amount of pigment concentration at each level of artificial hair color.

pinwheeling—Refers to coloring technique using vent brush producing a kaleidoscope of highlights.

porosity—The hair's ability to absorb liquid or moisture.

porous—Describes condition of cuticle when it is raised and open, allowing moisture and liquid to absorb.

powdered bleach—An alkaline product generally used in off-the-scalp bleach, which has less moisturizers in the formula than creme oil bleach.

predisposition test—See **patch test**.

prelighten—To first remove excess pigment from the hair. In two-step coloring, usually means lifting to one level lighter than target color.

presoften—Prepares resistant hair for better penetration of the hair color formula.

primary colors—In coloring, refers to the three basic colors of the color wheel, red, yellow, and blue, which make up all other colors when combined in different variations with one another.

processing lotion—A liquid, consisting of an extremely low percentage of hydrogen peroxide (often less than .5 of 1%) and thereby allowing for no oxidative action, which is used for mixing with semi or demi-permanent hair color.

progressive tint—Any hair dye that continues processing until removed, or gets darker with each application. Level System colors are considered nonprogressive.

protein—Groups of molecules created by combining amino acids; make up the most substance of the hair, skin, and nails.

psychological—Refers to the mental attitude of an individual.

Q

quaternary colors—Color combinations that are not primary, secondary, or tertiary.

R

regrowth—That portion of new growth near the scalp, which is untreated by color or chemicals.

repigmentizing—See **filler.**

result oriented—Putting more emphasis on the finished effect than the process by which it is achieved.

retouch—Application of color formula to the new growth of hair.

reverse frost—Tinting process that is actually corrective color. Adding or depositing color to lightened hair by means of the frosting technique (pulling hairs through a cap and applying darker color to selected strands). Usually requires filler to be effective.

rinses—Temporary colors that coat the cuticle of the hair and normally do not penetrate the cortex.

S

secondary colors—Colors created when pairs of primaries are mixed: Y + R = O, R + B = V, B + Y = G.

series—A category or grouping with similar attributes

shade—The degree of lightness and dark; it takes approximately *three shades* to equal *one level.*

Shade System—The system of permanent haircoloring using shade or tonal values as its standard for categorizing.

shading—The use of darker colors to create dimensional effects.

single-process—Haircoloring procedure that lifts and deposits in one application.

soap cap—Diluting remaining color formula (usually equal parts) with shampoo to prevent ends darkening with each application.

strand test—A sample formula applied to a small portion of hair to check expected results.

stripping shampoo—Formula for removing pigment from the hair to be lightened, for removing excess deposit from hair after tinting, or for helping presoftening.

subsection—The smaller divisions made within a section of hair, used for ultimate accuracy.

subtraction—Term used for lift or removal of pigment.

synthetic pigment—Color that is not natural to the structure of the hair. Usually derived from para-phenyldiamines.

T

target color—The desired end result of color

tea effect—Lightening of hair color due to high acidity of shampoos, rinses, or conditioners. Hair color is stripped from hair similar to the way tea lightens when lemon is added.

technician—Specialized professional dealing with exacting procedures and scientific information.

technique—Method, expertise, and style of color applications

temporary colors—Colors made from acid dyes readily removed by shampooing.

tenacity—The ability of the cuticle to resist penetration

tepid—Temperature of water between lukewarm and cool, unnoticeable when applied to the skin.

tertiary color—Color created when a primary is mixed with its neighboring secondary.

texture—Refers to the diameter of each shaft of hair. Usually categorized by fine, medium, or coarse.

theory—Scientific information that is supposed to work.

tint—Word used to describe hair color or the process of coloring hair. Refers also to the tonal cast of the hair.

tonal value—The value assigned to color that allows for description and distinction from another.

tone on tone (TNT)—Corresponding tones used for tinting in layers of color. Created by layering lightening formula over deposit color in random streaks or with foils.

twisters—Highlighting process that creates rippling lights on one-length hair.

V

vegetable dyes—Colors derived from plant sources.

virgin hair—Hair untreated by chemicals.

W

warm zone—The area of the hair shaft that develops tint more easily, within 1/2 inch of the scalp and body heat.

weave—Coloring technique using lighteners or deposit colors in which small amounts of hair are separated from subsections and tinted, then wrapped in foil or plastic to prevent leakage onto untinted hair. Currently the most popular and widespread method of off-the-scalp color.

working volume (WV)—The diluted volume of hydrogen peroxide resulting after mixing the color portion of the formula.

NOTES

NOTES

NOTES

NOTES

_____

_____

_____

_____

_____

_____

_____

_____

_____

_____

_____

_____

_____

_____

_____

_____

_____

_____

NOTES

NOTES